STRATEGIES, TECHNIQUES, APPROACHES & TO CRITICAL THINKING

A Clinical Reasoning Workbook for Nurses

5TH EDITION

STRATEGIES, TECHNIQUES, APPROACHES TO CRITICAL THINKING

A Clinical Reasoning Workbook for Nurses

Sandra Luz Martinez de Castillo, EdD, RN

Nursing Faculty
Contra Costa College
San Pablo, California

3251 Riverport Lane
St. Louis, MO 63043

STRATEGIES, TECHNIQUES, & APPROACHES TO CRITICAL THINKING:
A CLINICAL REASONING WORKBOOK FOR NURSES,
FIFTH EDITION

ISBN 978-1-4557-3390-3

Notices

Knowledge and best practice in this field are constantly changing. As new research and experience broaden our understanding, changes in research methods, professional practices, or medical treatment may become necessary. Practitioners and researchers must always rely on their own experience and knowledge in evaluating and using any information, methods, compounds, or experiments described herein. In using such information or methods they should be mindful of their own safety and the safety of others, including parties for whom they have a professional responsibility.

With respect to any drug or pharmaceutical products identified, readers are advised to check the most current information provided (i) on procedures featured or (ii) by the manufacturer of each product to be administered, to verify the recommended dose or formula, the method and duration of administration, and contraindications. It is the responsibility of practitioners, relying on their own experience and knowledge of their patients, to make diagnoses, to determine dosages and the best treatment for each individual patient, and to take all appropriate safety precautions.

To the fullest extent of the law, neither the Publisher nor the authors, contributors, or editors, assume any liability for any injury and/or damage to persons or property as a matter of products liability, negligence or otherwise, or from any use or operation of any methods, products, instructions, or ideas contained in the material herein.

ISBN 978-1-4557-3390-3

Executive Content Strategist: Lee Henderson
Senior Content Development Specialist: Rae L. Robertson
Content Coordinator: Kelly McGowan
Publishing Services Manager: Jeff Patterson
Senior Project Manager: Tracey Schriefer
Design Direction: Ashley Eberts

Printed in the United States of America.

Last digit is the print number: 9 8 7 6 5 4 3 2 1

PREFACE

Dear Nursing Student:

Nursing is an exciting and dynamic profession! It is a timeless profession that embraces the holistic nature of caring. To effectively address the health care needs of patients today, the professional nurse needs a strong knowledge base, practical clinical experience, critical thinking and clinical reasoning skills, and a commitment to continuous learning. The health care environment is changing, and new technological advances are shaping the work setting. Technology is not only a part of nursing practice with the incorporation of electronic medical records, but also a resource for obtaining continuous information. Used judiciously, technology can enhance the knowledge base and facilitate research activities that support evidence-based practice.

As a student, you will become familiar with the work done by the Quality and Safety Education for Nurses (QSEN) project in promoting the nursing core competencies of safety, evidence-based practice, teamwork and collaboration, patient-centered care, quality improvement, and informatics to improve the delivery of care. The clinical situations presented here will assist you to identify how one or more of these competencies are applied in clinical practice.

This manual is divided into seven sections. **Section One** focuses on building your knowledge base and applying this knowledge to short clinically based patient care situations. The clinical situations in Section One have three purposes: (1) to build your knowledge base and reinforce fundamental concepts and principles, (2) to demonstrate how learned knowledge is applied to clinical situations, and (3) to use critical thinking and clinical reasoning skills as you apply the Critical Thinking Model to the clinical situations. Remember that knowledge is fundamental to effectively using critical thinking skills and in promoting clinical reasoning. So, get actively involved in the knowledge building learning activities.

Section Two presents common clinical situations that will help you prioritize selected nursing interventions and make clinical decisions based on sound clinical reasoning. This section presents progressive clinical situations or unfolding clinical situations that allow you to see how nurses need to constantly assess and reevaluate patient care situations. Actively discussing the clinical situation with your peers and with your instructor provides an opportunity to hear other points of view, establish sound rationales, and reflect on your clinical decisions. The nursing process is included in this section to assist you to apply the components of assessment, nursing diagnosis, planning, and implementation.

Section Three presents clinical situations using the current handoff report format. You are asked to **analyze** and **interpret** the data based on the presenting clinical situation. Flow charts in the form of the patient's Nursing Care Rand/Kardex, Medication Record, Intake and Output Record, Nursing Notes, and History and Physical are provided to assist you in gathering further data. This activity helps you to (1) focus on gathering the data, both from the report and the flow charts; and (2) make relevant connections and synthesize the data. As in Section Two, unfolding clinical situations provide you with the opportunity to experience how patient situations change and thus require the nurse to apply critical thinking and clinical reasoning skills that promote the nursing competencies of safety and patient-centered care.

Section Four focuses on the development of management and leadership skills. As you begin to work with peers and to delegate to staff, work-related issues and personnel situations will arise. As with the patient care clinical situations, it is important to apply critical thinking skills as you work through the various clinical situations. Take time to discuss the clinical situation with your peers and focus on your management and leadership skills. Do you have a preferred style of management or leadership?

Section Five provides additional test questions for practice in selecting the most appropriate answer and making nursing decisions based on the clinical situations. You will draw from your knowledge base and your clinical experience as a nursing student to answer the test questions. Review and discuss your rationales, because this will continue to reinforce your knowledge base.

Section Six presents situations that assist you in beginning to apply leadership and delegation skills. The clinical situations offer you the opportunity to discuss the scope of practice of the registered nurse, the licensed vocational nurse, and unlicensed personnel as it relates to the situation. In addition, you will experience solving realistic work-related issues encountered in clinical practice.

Section Seven provides you the opportunity to use reference books and the Internet to research drugs while learning their side effects or adverse effects. Based on your research findings, it is important for you to compare and contrast drug information and further relate this information to patient teaching and follow-up care.

In addition, the following icon can be found on selected clinical situations. ⊖ This icon indicates that additional information can be accessed at the Evolve website at *http://evolve.elsevier.com/castillo/thinking*. For example, in Section One, under the Respiratory clinical situation, after accessing the web link you will hear audible breath sounds, and under the Pain Assessment clinical situation, you will be able to access various pain assessment scales in order to complete the clinical situation. The Delegation/Supervision icon ▤ highlights selected test questions and clinical situations that require you to consider the functions and duties of licensed and unlicensed personnel and make a decision that promotes patient safety. The Integrated Learning Activity icon ⚡ fosters the use of critical thinking and clinical reasoning skills. The Integrated Learning Activities promote discussion and consideration of patient status in selected unfolding clinical situations that require you to make clinical decisions.

Finally, as a beginning nursing student, you are encouraged to use the **Critical Thinking Model** to develop a process for working through patient care situations. The Critical Thinking Model will help you to apply critical thinking and clinical reasoning skills to make sound decisions. I hope that your passion for learning and for the nursing profession is enhanced by using these clinical situations!

Dr. Sandra Luz Martinez de Castillo

DEDICATION

To my parents, Blanca and Miguel, who instilled the value of education and service,
and to God for the many blessings and gifts.

REVIEWERS

Linda Grimsley, DSN, RN
Assistant Vice President for Academic Affairs
Associate Professor of Nursing
Albany State University
Albany, Georgia

Kristin Oneail, MSN, RN
Assistant Professor
Lourdes University
Sylvania, Ohio

Mary Lou Roark, MSN, RN
Nursing Instructor – ADN Program
Ashland Community and Technical College
Ashland, Kentucky

Mitchell J. Seal, RN-BC, EdD, MEd-IT, BSN, AS
Associate Director of Standards & Evaluation
Medical Education & Training Campus
Adjunct Faculty
University of the Incarnate Word
San Antonio, Texas

Deborah West, BSN
BSN Student
New York University
New York, New York

ACKNOWLEDGMENT

To all my nursing students—who foster my joy of teaching and learning . . .

CONTENTS

Section One—Knowledge Application

1-1   Professional Nursing Practice 1
1-2   Vital Signs 3
1-3   Temperature 5
1-4   Pulse 9
1-5   Respiration 13
1-6   Blood Pressure 17
1-7   Pain Assessment 21
1-8   Body Mechanics 23
1-9   Hygiene 25
1-10   Infection Control/Transmission of Organisms 27
1-11   Skin Integrity 31
1-12   Communication 35
1-13   Reporting Patient Status 39
1-14   Introduction to the Assessment Process 41
1-15   Basic Physical Assessment 43
1-16   Documentation 47
1-17   Self-Concept 49
1-18   Cultural Aspects of Nursing 51
1-19   Developing Culturally Competent Care 55
1-20   Introduction to Formulating a Nursing Diagnosis 57
1-21   Formulating a Nursing Diagnosis 59
1-22   Assessment of the Elderly Patient 63
1-23   Caring for the Surgical Patient 65
1-24   Wound Assessment 69
1-25   Wound Dressings 73
1-26   The Patient With Fluid and Electrolyte Imbalance 75
1-27   Elimination—Urinary 77
1-28   Elimination—Bowel 81
1-29   General Nutrition 83
1-30   Gastrointestinal Tract 85
1-31   Diabetes Mellitus 89
1-32   Complications of Diabetes Mellitus 93
1-33   Insulin Therapy 97
1-34   Legal Considerations in Nursing Practice 101
1-35   Review Questions 103

Section Two—Priority-Setting and Decision Making

2-1   Standards of Professional Performance 107
2-2   The Patient Undergoing Surgery 109
2-3   The Patient With an Intestinal Obstruction 113
2-4   The Patient With a Colostomy 117
2-5   The Patient With Colon Cancer 121
2-6   The Patient With Total Parenteral Nutrition 125
2-7   The Patient With Cirrhosis of the Liver 127
2-8   The Patient With Hepatic Encephalopathy 131
2-9   The Patient With Diabetes Mellitus 135
2-10   The Patient Undergoing Hemodialysis 139
2-11   The Patient With Peripheral Arterial Disease 143
2-12   The Patient With Chest Pain 145
2-13   The Patient With Heart Failure 147
2-14   The Patient With a Stroke 151
2-15   The Patient With Chronic Obstructive Pulmonary Disease 155

2-16 The Patient With a Chest Tube 159
2-17 The Patient With Urosepsis 163
2-18 The Patient With a Transurethral Resection of the Prostate 165
2-19 The Patient Receiving a Blood Transfusion 169
2-20 The Patient With Neutropenia 171
2-21 The Patient With a Hip Fracture 173
2-22 The Patient With a Fractured Tibia 177
2-23 The Patient With Cataract Surgery 179
2-24 The Patient With a Seizure Disorder 181
2-25 The Patient With a Do-Not-Rescuscitate Order 185
2-26 Legal Considerations 187

Section Three—Critical Thinking Model Application

3-1   Small Bowel Resection with Postop Care 189
3-2   Patient With GI Bleed and ETOH Abuse 191
3-3   Patient With Dehydration, Fever, Do-Not-Resuscitate Order 193
3-4   Patient With Fractured Tibia and Asthma 195
3-5   Patient With Pancreatitis and Central Line 197
3-6   Patient With a Head Trauma 199
3-7   Sensitive Postmortem Care 201
3-8   Patient Falling With Complications 203
3-9   Patient With Hypertension and Medication Error 205
3-10 Elderly Patient With MRSA 207
3-11 Patient With Viral Hepatitis 209
3-12 Patient With Prostate Cancer and Medication Error 211
3-13 Patient With Mastectomy and IV Fluid Overload 213
3-14 Patient With HF and Digoxin Toxicity 215
3-15 Patient With Hip Fracture and DVT 217
3-16 Patient Diagnosed With Pulmonary Embolus and on Anticoagulant Therapy 219
3-17 Patient With Signs and Symptoms of Postop Complications 221
3-18 Patient With Cellulitis Develops Angina 223
3-19 Patient With TURP and NS Irrigation 225
3-20 Patient With TAH and Epidural Catheter 227
3-21 Culturally Competent Nursing Care 229
3-22 Patient With Anthrax Exposure 231

Section Four—Management and Leadership

4-1   Mentoring and Nursing Management 233
4-2   Working Through the Change Process 235
4-3   Teamwork and Delegation 237
4-4   Practice and Ethical Issue 239
4-5   Teamwork and Collaboration 241
4-6   Advocating Cultural Competency and Sensitivity 243

Section Five—NCLEX Examination Preparation

5-1   NCLEX Examination Preparation #1 245
5-2   NCLEX Examination Preparation #2 247
5-3   NCLEX Examination Preparation #3 249
5-4   NCLEX Examination Preparation #4 251
5-5   NCLEX Examination Preparation #5 253
5-6   NCLEX Examination Preparation #6 255
5-7   NCLEX Examination Preparation #7 257
5-8   NCLEX Examination Preparation #8 259

Section Six—Professional Nursing Practice

6-1   Quality Nursing Practice Situation #1 (Postsurgical Patient) 261
6-2   Quality Nursing Practice Situation #2 (Caring and Advocacy) 263
6-3   Quality Nursing Practice Situation #3 (Adverse Client Outcome) 265

Section Seven—Evaluation

7-1   Working with Pharmacology #1 267
7-2   Working with Pharmacology #2 268
7-3   Working with Pharmacology #3 269
7-4   Working with Pharmacology #4 270
7-5   Working with Decision Making 271
7-6   Working with Priority Setting 272

Appendix A—List of Abbreviations

Appendix A—List of Abbreviations 273

Appendix B—List of Words and Phrases Commonly Used in the Book and Their Intended Meanings

Appendix B—List of Words and Phrases Commonly Used
              in the Book and Their Intended Meanings 274

1-1 PROFESSIONAL NURSING PRACTICE

Fill in the blanks with the requested information:

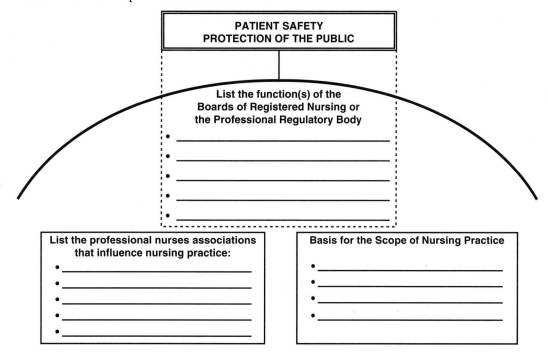

PATIENT SAFETY
PROTECTION OF THE PUBLIC

List the function(s) of the
Boards of Registered Nursing or
the Professional Regulatory Body

- _____
- _____
- _____
- _____
- _____

List the professional nurses associations
that influence nursing practice:

- _____
- _____
- _____
- _____
- _____

Basis for the Scope of Nursing Practice

- _____
- _____
- _____
- _____

CLINICAL SITUATION   A student nurse started clinical practice in the acute care setting. The assignment includes caring for a client who will be transferred to a skilled nursing facility today but needs morning care, bathing, and assistance with feeding before discharge. The client also has an indwelling urinary catheter.

Pertinent Terminology	Definition
Nurse Practice Act	_____
Scope of Nursing Practice	_____
Independent Nursing Functions	_____
Dependent Nursing Functions	_____
Interdependent Nursing Functions	_____

From the clinical situation, identify the type of nursing function for the following interventions:

Assigned Nursing Care	Function
Morning care, bathing, feeding, indwelling urinary catheter care	☐ Independent ☐ Dependent ☐ Interdependent

The family arrives and asks whether their father will be transferred to the skilled facility with the urinary catheter. The student consults with the RN, who says that "it should probably be removed."

Assigned Nursing Care	Function
Urinary catheter removal	☐ Independent ☐ Dependent ☐ Interdependent

The RN and the student return to the client's room. The RN is getting ready to administer the morning medications to the client.

Assigned Nursing Care	Function
Administration of medication	☐ Independent ☐ Dependent ☐ Interdependent

The RN is caring for another patient who had abdominal surgery 3 days ago. The patient asks the RN when the urinary catheter is to be removed. The nurse refers to the standard protocol for urinary catheter removal for postoperative patients that is approved by the agency.

Assigned Nursing Care	Function
Urinary catheter removal postoperative based on standard protocol	☐ Independent ☐ Dependent ☐ Interdependent

Integrated Learning Activity: With a partner, connect to website of the State Board of Registered Nursing or the professional regulatory body for your state and review the regulations governing the scope of practice for the following situations.

1. What is the position of the State Board of Registered Nursing or the professional regulatory body of the state regarding services provided by student nurses?

2. What is the position of the State Board of Registered Nursing or the professional regulatory body of the state regarding delegation of tasks?

1-2 VITAL SIGNS

List the common routes for taking a **temperature:**

1. _____

2. _____

3. _____

4. _____

5. _____

The **blood pressure** may be auscultated in the

_____ and _____ spaces.

Use the diagram to identify the **pulse sites** in the body.

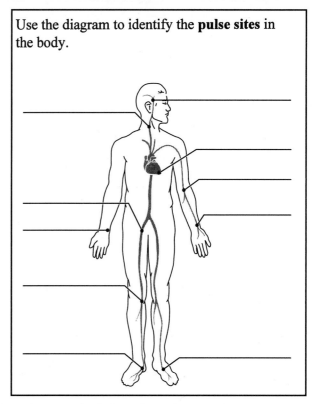

CLINICAL SITUATION   An adult male client has been having a high fever for 2 days. At the physician's office he was found to be febrile. Additionally, the client is complaining of chills, night sweats, anorexia, and fatigue. He is admitted to the hospital. The physician's orders include vital signs (VS) every 4 hours. On admission he had pyrexia. The admission VS are T 102.4° F, P 96, R 26, BP 148/88, pulse ox 98%, pain level 0.

Pertinent Terminology	Definition
Vital Signs	_____
Temperature	_____
Pulse	_____
Respiration	_____
Pulse Oximetry (Pulse Ox)	_____
Blood Pressure	_____
Febrile	_____
Pyrexia	_____
Anorexia	_____
Fatigue	_____

From the clinical situation, record today's date and the 0800 admission VS on the following **Graphic Sheet.** Enter the following vital signs for today:

1200	T 103.6° F,	P 108,	R 32,	BP 160/76,	Pulse ox 97%
1600	T 101.2° F,	P 98,	R 28,	BP 154/82,	Pulse ox 96%
2000	T 100.0° F,	P 80,	R 24,	BP 150/90,	Pulse ox 98%

Record the 0800 VS for the next day: T 99.6° F, P 72, R 18, BP 146/94, Pulse ox 97%

Draw a line between the temperature recordings to create a graph.

GRAPHIC SHEET

Date												
Time	0400	0800	1200	1600	2000	2400	0400	0800	1200	1600	2000	2400
40° C 104° F												
39.4° C 103° F												
38.9° C 102° F												
38.3° C 101° F												
37.7° C 100° F												
37.2° C 99° F												
37 36.6° C 98° F												
36.1° C 97° F												
35.5° C 96° F												
Pulse												
Resp.												
B/P												
SpO$_2$												

Integrated Learning Activity: With a partner, identify the normal range(s) for the VS in the adult.

Body temperature **Oral**   _____

Axillary   _____

_____

Rectal   _____

_____

Tympanic   _____

Pulse   _____

Respirations   _____

Blood pressure   _____

Pulse oximetry   _____

Pain assessment   _____

1-3 TEMPERATURE

The **body temperature** is regulated through the

_____ .

Body temperature is affected by:

1. _____

2. _____

3. _____

4. _____

5. _____

6. _____

Body temperature remains constant through **heat production** and **heat loss.**

Factors that influence heat production:

- _____
- _____

Factors that influence heat loss:

- _____
- _____
- _____
- _____

CLINICAL SITUATION   A 79-year-old client was brought to the emergency department after having fainted while sitting outside at a family gathering. The physician admitted the client with the diagnosis of heat-stroke. On admission the vital signs are T 40.5° C, P 100, R 26, BP 118/64. The client's skin is flushed and feels hot and dry. The client is awake, denies pain but is complaining of nausea. The physician orders the temperature to be monitored every hour.

Pertinent Terminology	Definition
Temperature	_____
Core Temperature	_____
Hyperthermia	_____
Hypothermia	_____
Heatstroke	_____
Conduction	_____
Convection	_____
Evaporation	_____
Radiation	_____

From the clinical situation, explain how the **evaporation factor initially** acts to prevent the client from developing heatstroke:

_____

Fill in the thermometers to reflect the temperature readings (both Celsius and Fahrenheit) for your shift.

Time	Reading	Non-mercury Thermometer
0900	39.8° C	
1000	40.1° C	
1100	38.7° C	
1200	103.8° F	
1300	102.6° F	
1400	101.4° F	
1500	100.2° F	

✏ **Integrated Learning Activity: Graph** the temperature readings for your shift. Draw a line between each temperature recording. Compare your **Temperature Recording Sheet** with that of a partner.

Temperature Recording Sheet

Time	0800	0900	1000	1100	1200	1300	1400	1500
40.5° C 105° F								
40° C 104° F								
39.4° C 103° F								
38.9° C 102° F								
38.3° C 101° F								
37.7° C 100° F								
37.2° C 99° F								
37 36.6° C 98° F								
36.1° C 97° F								
35.5° C 96° F								

APPLYING CRITICAL THINKING TO TEST QUESTIONS

INSTRUCTIONS: Circle the one best answer for each test question. Write your rationale for selecting the answer. To enhance your learning and test-taking skills, discuss your answer and rationale with a partner. The answer and the rationale can be found on the back of this page.

1. The nurse is using a digital thermometer to take an oral temperature. After taking the oral temperature, the nurse obtains a reading of 94.2° F. Which follow-up action is most appropriate for the nurse to do?
   a. Use another digital thermometer to retake the temperature.
   b. Feel the client's skin temperature.
   c. Take a rectal temperature.
   d. Document the findings.

   Rationale for your selection: _____
   _____
   _____
   _____
   _____
   _____

2. The nurse obtains an axillary temperature of 97.4° F on a client. In graphing the temperature, it is most appropriate for the nurse to:
   a. write "see nurse's notes" above the temperature reading.
   b. identify the temperature reading with an "Ax."
   c. graph the oral equivalent temperature of 98.4° F.
   d. just graph 97.4° F on the form.

   Rationale for your selection: _____
   _____
   _____
   _____
   _____
   _____

3. The nurse is caring for a client who has an oral temperature of 99.6° F at 8:00 AM, the start of the day shift. The client's care plan indicates that vital signs should be taken once a shift. In planning care for the client, which action is most appropriate?
   a. Ensure that the temperature is taken promptly at 4:00 PM.
   b. Call the physician for a more frequent order.
   c. Take the temperature as necessary.
   d. Begin cooling measures.

   Rationale for your selection: _____
   _____
   _____
   _____
   _____
   _____

ANSWER KEY FOR
APPLYING CRITICAL THINKING SKILLS TO TEST QUESTIONS

HELPFUL HINTS: Read all test questions carefully. Identify key words in the question that will guide you in answering the question. In these test questions the **key words** to consider are **"follow-up"** and **"most appropriate."** Compare your rationale with the one in the test question.

1. The nurse is using a digital thermometer to take an oral temperature. After taking the oral temperature, the nurse obtains a reading of 94.2° F. Which follow-up action is most appropriate for the nurse to do?
   a. Use another digital thermometer to retake the temperature.
   b. Feel the client's skin temperature.
   c. Take a rectal temperature.
   d. Document the findings.

   Rationale: The answer is (a). Because the nurse is using a digital thermometer, it is important for the nurse to ensure that the equipment is functioning. The temperature recording is low and should be taken again. Option (b) does not provide the most accurate information, and (c) is not appropriate; option (d) should be done after the temperature is verified.

2. The nurse obtains an axillary temperature of 97.4° F on a client. In graphing the temperature, it is most appropriate for the nurse to:
   a. write "see nurse's notes" above the temperature reading.
   b. identify the temperature reading with an "Ax."
   c. graph the oral equivalent temperature of 98.4° F.
   d. just graph 97.4° F on the form.

   Rationale: The answer is (b). It is important for the nurse to identify the appropriate information on where the temperature was taken. Options (a), (c), and (d) do not accurately document the temperature information.

3. The nurse is caring for a client who has an oral temperature of 99.6° F at 8:00 AM, the start of the day shift. The client's care plan indicates that vital signs should be taken once a shift. In planning care for the client, which action is most appropriate?
   a. Ensure that the temperature is taken promptly at 4:00 PM.
   b. Call the physician for a more frequent order.
   c. Take the temperature as necessary.
   d. Begin cooling measures.

   Rationale: The answer is (c). The nurse can make an independent decision to take the temperature more frequently to ensure safe nursing care. Option (a) does not allow for a thorough, ongoing assessment. Options (b) and (d) are not necessary at this time.

1-4 PULSE

The normal **pulse rate range** for an adult is:

_____.

The **pulse characteristics** include a description
of the _____, _____, and
_____ of the pulse.

The **pulse** is affected by:

1. _____
2. _____
3. _____
4. _____
5. _____
6. _____
7. _____
8. _____

Draw circles on the diagram that identify the
sites where the **pulse** is found in the body.

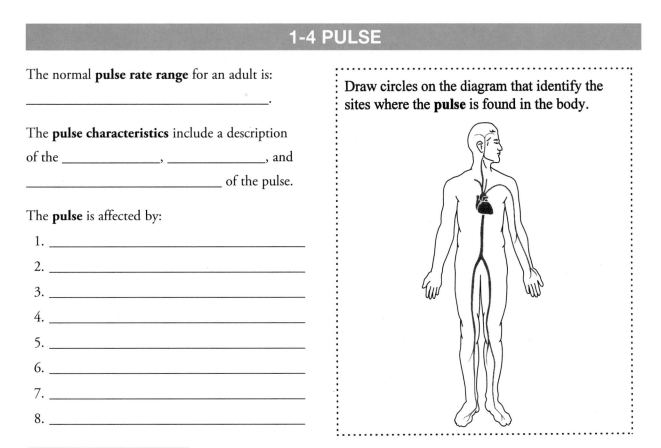

CLINICAL SITUATION   A 52-year-old male client has been complaining of a rapid heartbeat. He says
that it feels as if his "heart is racing." His wife took him to the urgent care clinic where he was found to have an
irregular pulse of 160 bpm; he was transferred to the hospital. On admission to the hospital his vital signs are
T 98.4° F, P 168, R 28, BP 146/90, denies pain. His skin is moist and he is very anxious. The physician orders
the administration of cardiac medications and orders the pulse to be monitored every 2 hours.

Pertinent Terminology	Definition
Pulse	_____
	_____
Peripheral Pulse	_____
Apical Pulse	_____
Stroke Volume	_____
Cardiac Output	_____
	_____
Pulse Rhythm	_____
Pulse Quality	_____
Tachycardia	_____
Bradycardia	_____
Arrhythmia	_____
Pulse Deficit	_____

From the clinical situation, use the admission pulse of 168 bpm to assist in identifying the words in the parenthesis that would **best describe** the characteristics of this pulse:

Pulse Characteristic	Descriptive Words	Selected Word(s)
Rate	(rapid, tachycardia, bradycardia, increased)	
Rhythm	(regular, irregular, abnormal, dysrhythmia)	
Quality	(weak, thready, bounding, difficult to palpate)	

Integrated Learning Activity: With a partner, identify the **pulse site** in each diagram and **write in the reason** for checking the pulse from this area.

Pulse: _____

Reason:_____
_____

Pulse: _____

Reason:_____
_____

Pulse: _____

Reason:_____
_____
_____

Pulse: _____

Reason:_____
_____
_____

The **apical pulse** is taken when _____
_____.

To take an **apical pulse,** the stethoscope is placed on _____
_____.

APPLYING CRITICAL THINKING SKILLS TO TEST QUESTIONS

INSTRUCTIONS: Circle the one best answer for each test question. Write your rationale for selecting the answer. To enhance your learning and test-taking skills, discuss your answer and rationale with a partner. The answer and the rationale can be found on the back of this page.

1. The nurse describes the radial pulse as "thready and irregular" after taking morning vital signs. The most appropriate follow-up nursing action is to:
   a. notify the physician.
   b. check the apical pulse.
   c. graph the pulse.
   d. check the previous pulse.

   Rationale for your selection: _____
   _____
   _____
   _____
   _____
   _____

2. The nurse is auscultating the apical pulse on a client. In counting the apical pulse, the nurse counts:
   a. each lub-dub as one beat.
   b. each lub-dub as two beats.
   c. the pulse for 10 seconds and multiplies by 6.
   d. the pulse for 30 seconds and multiplies by 2.

   Rationale for your selection: _____
   _____
   _____
   _____
   _____
   _____

3. The nurse is instructed to check for a pedal pulse on a client at the beginning of the shift. To carry out this intervention, it is most appropriate for the nurse to:
   a. count the brachial pulse for 30 seconds.
   b. count the posterior tibial pulse for 1 full minute.
   c. palpate for the dorsalis pedis.
   d. palpate for the popliteal pulse.

   Rationale for your selection: _____
   _____
   _____
   _____
   _____
   _____

ANSWER KEY FOR
APPLYING CRITICAL THINKING SKILLS TO TEST QUESTIONS

HELPFUL HINTS: Read all test questions carefully. Identify key words in the question that will guide you in answering the question. In these test questions the **key words** to consider are **"most appropriate."** Compare your rationale with the one in the test question.

1. The nurse describes the radial pulse as "thready and irregular" after taking morning vital signs. The most appropriate follow-up nursing action is to:
   a. notify the physician.
   b. check the apical pulse.
   c. graph the pulse.
   d. check the previous pulse.

   Rationale: The answer is (b). It is the nurse's responsibility to validate abnormal findings. Therefore, the most appropriate follow-up action in this question is to check the apical pulse. This will assist the nurse to fully assess the findings. Although options (a), (c), and (d) are actions that the nurse would do, they are not the most appropriate for this situation.

2. The nurse is auscultating the apical pulse on a client. In counting the apical pulse, the nurse counts:
   a. each lub-dub as one beat.
   b. each lub-dub as two beats.
   c. the pulse for 10 seconds and multiplies by 6.
   d. the pulse for 30 seconds and multiplies by 2.

   Rationale: The answer is (a). Each lub represents the closure of the mitral and tricuspid valves during systole and the dub represents the closure of the aortic and pulmonic valves during diastole. Together the lub-dub sounds are counted as one beat. Options (b), (c), and (d) do not describe the correct technique for counting the apical pulse.

3. The nurse is instructed to check for a pedal pulse on a client at the beginning of the shift. To carry out this intervention, it is most appropriate for the nurse to:
   a. count the brachial pulse for 30 seconds.
   b. count the posterior tibial pulse for 1 full minute.
   c. palpate for the dorsalis pedis.
   d. palpate for the popliteal pulse.

   Rationale: The answer is (c). This question addresses the nurse's understanding of pedal pulses. Therefore, in this situation, it is most appropriate for the nurse to locate and palpate the pulse in the feet. Although option (b) identifies one of the pedal pulses, it is not necessary to take a pedal pulse for a full minute. Options (a) and (d) are not appropriate in carrying out this nursing order.

1-5 RESPIRATION

The normal respiration rate range for an adult is _____.
The **characteristics of respiration** include a description of the _____, _____, and _____ of the respirations.
The factors that affect the **characteristics of the respiration** include:

1. _____
2. _____
3. _____
4. _____
5. _____
6. _____
7. _____
8. _____
9. _____
10. _____

A **normal** respiratory pattern consists of a full inspiration and a full expiration counted over one minute as the diagram illustrates:

The diagram demonstrates a _____ respiratory pattern.

The diagram demonstrates a _____ respiratory pattern.

CLINICAL SITUATION   A male client has been a smoker for 20 years. He has noticed increased shortness of breath (SOB) for the past 6 months and is complaining of a productive cough with thick whitish phlegm. The nurse notices that his respiratory rate is 32 and regular and describes his lung sounds as fine crackling sounds heard on inspiration. Pulse oximetry is 92% on room air.

Pertinent Terminology	Definition
Respiration	
Tachypnea	
Bradypnea	
Eupnea	
Apnea	
Orthopnea	
Dyspnea	
Cheyne-Stokes	
Kussmaul	
Phlegm	

From the clinical situation, use the respiratory rate of 32 to assist in identifying the words in the parenthesis that would **best describe** the characteristics of this respiratory pattern:

Respiratory Characteristic	Descriptive Words	Selected Word(s)
Rate	(eupnea, tachypnea, bradypnea, apnea)	
Depth	(deep, full inspiration/expiration, short, shallow)	
Rhythm	(regular, irregular)	

Ⓔ **Draw a line** to match the **identified lung sounds** below with the appropriate description. (Visit *www.evolve.elsevier.com/castillo* to hear sample lung sounds.)

Wheeze   crackling sound, may be fine or coarse, heard frequently on inspiration

Crackle   coarse, harsh, loud sound, best heard on expiration

Gurgle   continuous high-pitched musical sound best heard on expiration

Circle the lung sound that best describes the client's lung sounds.

⚡ **Integrated Learning Activity:** Draw a diagram that represents the respiratory pattern identified under each box. Compare and discuss your diagrams with a partner.

```
┌─────────────────────────────┐     ┌─────────────────────────────┐
│  ┌───────────────────────┐  │     │  ┌───────────────────────┐  │
│  │                       │  │     │  │                       │  │
│  │                       │  │     │  │                       │  │
│  └───────────────────────┘  │     │  └───────────────────────┘  │
│  1 minute                   │     │  1 minute                   │
│                             │     │                             │
│  Respiration Pattern: Apnea │     │  Respiration Pattern: Tachypnea │
│                             │     │                             │
│  ┌───────────────────────┐  │     │  ┌───────────────────────┐  │
│  │                       │  │     │  │                       │  │
│  │                       │  │     │  │                       │  │
│  └───────────────────────┘  │     │  └───────────────────────┘  │
│  1 minute                   │     │  1 minute                   │
│                             │     │                             │
│  Respiration Pattern: Cheyne-Stokes │  Respiration Pattern: Kussmaul │
└─────────────────────────────┘     └─────────────────────────────┘
```

APPLYING CRITICAL THINKING SKILLS TO TEST QUESTIONS

INSTRUCTIONS: Circle the best answer for each test question. Write your rationale for selecting the answer. To enhance your learning and test-taking skills, discuss your answer and rationale with a partner. The answer and the rationale can be found on the back of this page.

1. The nurse is taking the vital signs of a client who has shortness of breath. In counting the respiratory rate it is most important for the nurse to:
   a. observe the rise and fall of the chest for 15 seconds.
   b. assess the respiratory pattern for 30 seconds.
   c. sit the client in a semi-Fowler position.
   d. count the respiratory rate for 1 minute.

   Rationale for your selection: _____
   _____
   _____
   _____
   _____
   _____

2. The nurse assesses the respiratory rate of an adult client to be 20 and unlabored. The most appropriate follow-up nursing intervention is to:
   a. reassess the respiratory rate.
   b. graph the findings.
   c. check the pulse oximeter.
   d. place the client in high Fowler position.

   Rationale for your selection: _____
   _____
   _____
   _____
   _____
   _____

3. The physician orders pulse oximetry checks on the client once a shift. To effectively use the pulse oximeter on the client, the nurse would:
   a. place the pulse oximeter on the client's finger and wait for a reading.
   b. give the client oxygen before using the pulse oximeter.
   c. place the client in high Fowler position.
   d. use the pulse oximeter only when the client has dyspnea.

   Rationale for your selection: _____
   _____
   _____
   _____
   _____
   _____

ANSWER KEY FOR
APPLYING CRITICAL THINKING SKILLS TO TEST QUESTIONS

HELPFUL HINTS: Read all test questions carefully. Identify key words in the question that will guide you in answering the question. In these test questions the **key words** to consider are **"most important," "most appropriate,"** and **"effectively use."** Compare your rationale with the one found for each question.

1. The nurse is taking the vital signs of a client who has shortness of breath. In counting the respiratory rate it is most important for the nurse to:
   a. observe the rise and fall of the chest for 15 seconds.
   b. assess the respiratory pattern for 30 seconds.
   c. sit the client in a semi-Fowler position.
   d. count the respiratory rate for 1 minute.

   Rationale: The answer is (d). Because the client has shortness of breath, it is most important for the nurse to fully assess the respirations for 1 minute. Option (a) does not allow the nurse to fully assess the respiratory pattern; option (b) assessment of an abnormal respiratory pattern should be done for 1 full minute, and option (c) compromises the respiratory system.

2. The nurse assesses the respiratory rate of an adult client to be 20 and unlabored. The most appropriate follow-up nursing intervention is to:
   a. reassess the respiratory rate.
   b. graph the findings.
   c. check the pulse oximeter.
   d. place the client in high Fowler position.

   Rationale: The answer is (b). The findings are normal; therefore, the next nursing intervention is to graph the findings. Options (a), (c), and (d) can be performed if the nurse assesses an abnormal rate.

3. The physician orders pulse oximetry checks on the client once a shift. To effectively use the pulse oximeter on the client, the nurse would:
   a. place the pulse oximeter on the client's finger and wait for a reading.
   b. give the client oxygen before using the pulse oximeter.
   c. place the client in high Fowler position.
   d. use the pulse oximeter only when the client has dyspnea.

   Rationale: The answer is (a). The answer describes how to use the pulse oximeter. Options (b) and (c) are incorrect in answering how to effectively use the pulse oximeter. Option (d) is incorrect: a pulse oximeter can be used to assess oxygenation in any client.

1-6 BLOOD PRESSURE

The normal blood pressure for an

adult is _____.

Factors that affect the blood pressure include:

1. _____
2. _____
3. _____
4. _____
5. _____
6. _____
7. _____
8. _____
9. _____
10. _____

Identify the parts of the following items used in obtaining a blood pressure:

CLINICAL SITUATION   A 65-year-old African-American man goes weekly to the hypertension clinic for blood pressure checks. He has a 20-year history of smoking 2 packs of cigarettes a day. His father died from heart disease and his brother has hypertension. He lives alone, does not get out much and his diet is mainly premade frozen meals or canned foods. His current blood pressure reading is 174/104 mm Hg, and he is complaining of a headache and dizziness when getting up in the morning.

Pertinent Terminology	Definition
Blood Pressure	
Systolic Pressure	
Diastolic Pressure	
Korotkoff Sounds	
Pulse Pressure	
Prehypertension	
Hypertension	
Hypotension	
Orthostatic Hypotension	
Auscultatory Gap	

From the clinical situation, identify the **factors** that predisposed the patient for development of hypertension:

_____   _____   _____

_____   _____   _____

The clinic nurse monitors the patient's blood pressure for 3 days:

Day 1	
11:00 AM	210/110
11:15 AM	202/104
11:30 AM	190/98

Day 2	
11:00 AM	188/100
11:15 AM	170/98
11:30 AM	164/94

Day 3—11:00 AM	
Lying	178/100
Sitting	166/90
Standing	150/90

⚡ **Integrated Learning Activity:** Record the blood pressure readings on the flow sheet using the symbol "**V**" to identify the systolic reading and the symbol "**Λ**" for the diastolic reading. Connect both symbols with a straight line. Identify the orthostatic blood pressure readings with the appropriate symbols. Compare your flow sheet with a partner.

Blood Pressure Flow Sheet

Date	Day 1			Day 2			Day 3		
Time	11:00	11:15	11:30	11:00	11:15	11:30	11:00		
240									
230									
220									
210									
200									
190									
180									
170									
160									
150									
140									
130									
120									
110									
100									
90									
80									
70									

APPLYING CRITICAL THINKING SKILLS TO TEST QUESTIONS

INSTRUCTIONS: Circle the one best answer for each test question. Write your rationale for selecting the answer. To enhance your learning and test-taking skills, discuss your answer and rationale with a partner. The answer and the rationale can be found on the back of this page.

1. The nurse is preparing to take the blood pressure of an adult patient for the first time. After placing the cuff on the patient's upper arm, it is most important for the nurse to:
   a. wait 1 minute before taking the blood pressure.
   b. place the stethoscope at the antecubital space.
   c. inflate the cuff to 150 mm Hg.
   d. palpate the systolic pressure.

   Rationale for your selection: _____
   _____
   _____
   _____
   _____
   _____

2. The nurse uses a Doppler device to obtain the blood pressure measurement. In documenting the findings, the nurse will record the:
   a. systolic measurement.
   b. systolic and diastolic measurements.
   c. diastolic measurement.
   d. auscultatory gap.

   Rationale for your selection: _____
   _____
   _____
   _____
   _____
   _____

3. In which of the following clients would the nurse expect a decreased blood pressure? A client:
   a. who is very anxious about being in the hospital.
   b. scheduled for major surgery.
   c. with a severe head injury.
   d. who hemorrhaged after surgery.

   Rationale for your selection: _____
   _____
   _____
   _____
   _____
   _____

ANSWER KEY FOR
APPLYING CRITICAL THINKING SKILLS TO TEST QUESTIONS

HELPFUL HINTS: Read all test questions carefully. Identify key words in the question that will guide you in answering the question. In these test questions the key words to consider are **"first time," "initial action,"** and **"most appropriate."** Compare your rationale with the one in the test question.

1. The nurse is preparing to take the blood pressure of an adult patient for the first time. After placing the cuff on the patient's upper arm, it is most important for the nurse to:
   a. wait 1 minute before taking the blood pressure.
   b. place the stethoscope at the antecubital space.
   c. inflate the cuff to 150 mm Hg.
   d. palpate the systolic pressure.

   Rationale: The answer is (d). Palpating for the systolic pressure provides the nurse with information for inflating the cuff to ensure an accurate systolic reading. Although option (b) is an action that the nurse would do, it is not the initial action. Options (a) and (c) are not appropriate for this situation.

2. The nurse uses a Doppler device to obtain the blood pressure measurement. In documenting the findings, the nurse will record the:
   a. systolic measurement.
   b. systolic and diastolic measurements.
   c. diastolic measurement.
   d. auscultatory gap.

   Rationale: The answer is (a). Doppler devices amplify sounds. In finding the blood pressure, only the systolic measurement can be obtained with the use of a Doppler device. Options (b), (c), and (d) are not possible options when using a Doppler device.

3. In which of the following clients would the nurse expect a decreased blood pressure? A client:
   a. who is very anxious about being in the hospital.
   b. scheduled for major surgery.
   c. with a severe head injury.
   d. who hemorrhaged after surgery.

   Rationale: The answer is (d). Conditions that decrease the blood volume also decrease the cardiac output, which contributes to a decrease in blood pressure. Options (a), (b), and (c) are conditions that cause vasoconstriction, which increases the blood pressure.

1-7 PAIN ASSESSMENT

Pain is the _____ vital sign.

Assessment of the patient's pain is done:

_____

_____

_____

Common behaviors that may indicate that the patient is experiencing pain include:

1. _____

2. _____

3. _____

4. _____

5. _____

List **words** frequently used by patients to describe the quality of the pain sensation.

CLINICAL SITUATION   Patient A is a 27-year-old male who sustained a sprained left ankle 2 days ago after tripping and falling while playing basketball.

Patient B is a 56-year-old female who is diagnosed with bone cancer and is admitted to the hospital for chemotherapy.

Patient C is a 79-year-old female who had a right hip replacement 2 days ago. She continues to demonstrate disorientation to time and place as noted on admission to the hospital. However, the handoff report indicates that she showed signs of increased restlessness during the night and this morning.

Pertinent Terminology	Definition
Pain	_____
Acute Pain	_____
Chronic Pain	_____
Pain Threshold	_____
Pain Tolerance	_____
Pain Assessment Tool	_____

UNIDIMENSIONAL PAIN ASSESSMENT SCALES

Visit *www.evolve.elsevier.com/castillo* to access the various pain assessment scales. **Select the most appropriate pain scale** for the patients in the clinical situation.

- For Patient A, the _____ pain assessment scale is appropriate for the nurse to use.

- For Patient B, the _____ pain assessment scale is appropriate for the nurse to use.

- For Patient C, the _____ assessment scales are appropriate for the nurse to use.

Use the clinical situation and these follow-up assessments to make clinical decisions that focus on **patient-centered care** and **pain management.**

On assessing Patient A at 0800, the patient reports a pain level of 5. The swelling from the left ankle has remained the same since the injury. His pain medication is ordered q4h and the last dose was given at 0415. The most appropriate follow-up is to _____

_____

On assessing Patient B at 0815, the patient reports a pain level of 9. The patient has a PCA with continuous morphine sulfate infusion. Morphine sulfate 3 mg is ordered q2h direct IV injection for breakthrough pain. It was last given at 0530. The most appropriate follow-up is to _____

_____

On assessing Patient C at 0745, the nurse finds the patient restless, grabbing at her bed linens, and pulling on her right hip dressing. The nurse is unable to obtain a verbal pain level from the patient. The most appropriate follow-up is to _____

_____

Integrated Learning Activity: With a partner, read and evaluate the following statements. Decide whether the statement is True or False. For each statement, provide a rationale that supports your clinical decision.

Statement	True	False	Rationale to Support Your Clinical Decision
Changes in pulse, respirations, and blood pressure are strong indicators of the intensity of pain experienced by the patient.			_____ _____ _____ _____
Older adults report pain less often.			_____ _____ _____ _____
Self-report of pain level is the most reliable method to assess pain intensity.			_____ _____ _____ _____

1-8 BODY MECHANICS

List the **factors** that affect a patient's ability to move and maintain body alignment:

1. _____

2. _____

3. _____

4. _____

5. _____

6. _____

7. _____

Use the diagram to identify the **four basic principles** of body mechanics:

1. _____

2. _____

3. _____

4. _____

CLINICAL SITUATION   The client has had a cerebral vascular accident (CVA) and as a result has left-sided hemiplegia. The physician orders the client to be out of bed (OOB) twice a day and to be turned every 2 hours while in bed. The RN asks the staff to do passive range of motion (ROM) exercises to the client's left side and to use supportive devices to ensure proper body alignment. The client is to be encouraged to do active ROM on the right side extremities.

Pertinent Terminology	Definition
Range of Motion	
Active ROM	
Passive ROM	
CVA	
Hemiplegia	
Alignment	
Hand Roll	
Trochanter Roll	
Foot Board	
Plantar Flexion	
Flaccid	

From the clinical situation, **(1) identify** the **major body areas** that would require special nursing care, **(2) select** the most appropriate **supportive device** from the list that will assist in maintaining proper body alignment for the client, and **(3) state the complication** the nursing care will help to prevent.

Hand roll	Trochanter roll	Pillow	Trapeze bar	Footboard

Major Body Area	Supportive Device	This Helps to Prevent

Select the activities of daily living (ADLs) below that the client can perform **independently** throughout the day that encourage **active ROM** to the **right side** of the body:

- ☐ Brushing teeth
- ☐ Transferring OOB
- ☐ Flexing/extending ankle
- ☐ Combing hair

- ☐ Ambulating
- ☐ Standing
- ☐ Washing face
- ☐ Feeding

Integrated Learning Activity: With a partner, beginning with number 1, **number the following interventions** in the order necessary to assist the client to transfer from the bed to a wheelchair:

_____   Place wheelchair at a 45-degree angle to the bed.

_____   Lock the wheelchair brakes.

_____   Assist the client to a sitting position at the side of the bed.

_____   Provide instructions to the client.

_____   Cross left lower extremity over right lower extremity.

_____   Have the client pivot toward the wheelchair.

_____   Lower the client into the wheelchair.

_____   Stand the client; support left lower extremity.

_____   Have the client support left upper extremity with right upper extremity.

1-9 HYGIENE

The **purpose of providing a bath** is to:

1. _____

2. _____

3. _____

4. _____

5. _____

Identify the various types of baths:

1. _____

2. _____

3. _____

4. _____

Place a "✔" mark on the information that best describes the following.

Early morning care includes:

☐ Starting the bath early in the morning.

☐ Providing/assisting with oral hygiene.

☐ Washing face and hands.

☐ Offering bedpan, urinal, or assisting to the bathroom.

Hour of sleep care includes:

☐ Providing a back rub for the client.

☐ Straightening the bed linens.

☐ Providing/assisting with oral hygiene.

☐ Taking the vital signs.

CLINICAL SITUATION   An 88-year-old female client has been in the hospital for 2 days with an irregular heartbeat. She is confused and just lies in bed. The RN informs you that the client has urinary and bowel incontinence and is wearing an adult incontinence pad. Her skin is very fragile, she has several ecchymotic areas on the lower extremities, she is wearing antiembolic stockings, and the pneumatic compression stockings are off. Her toenails are long, yellowish, and thick. She has dried feces under her fingernails.

Pertinent Terminology	Definition
Antiembolic Stockings	_____
	_____
Pneumatic Compression Stockings	_____
Stomatitis	_____
	_____
Canthus	_____
	_____
Ecchymosis	_____
	_____
Perineum	_____
	_____
Labia Majora	_____
	_____
Labia Minora	_____
	_____
Prepuce	_____
	_____

Use the clinical situation to identify the **most appropriate** nursing interventions for taking care of the client's hands and feet. **Circle** the nursing interventions below that you would implement:

NURSING INTERVENTIONS

Hands

1. Do nothing until the RN informs you.
2. Soak the hands in lukewarm water.
3. Give the bath as usual, but do not soak the hands.
4. Use a greenstick or cotton swab to remove the feces.
5. Cut the fingernails carefully to prevent further collection under the nail beds.

Feet

1. Remove the antiembolic stockings during the bath.
2. Clean the feet with lukewarm water.
3. Give a partial bath; apply lotion.
4. Dry well between the toes.
5. Cut the toenails carefully straight across.

Describe the proper method for performing perineal care on a:

Female: _____

_____

Male: _____

_____

⚡ **Integrated Learning Activity:** With a partner, identify the type of bath **most appropriate** for the following clinical situations:

Clinical Situations	Type of Bath		
A 39-year-old woman who had abdominal surgery 5 days ago and will be discharged this morning	Complete	Partial Self-help	Shower (MD order/ policy)
A 56-year-old patient admitted with lung problems who gets very short of breath with mild exertion	Complete	Partial	Shower
A 23-year-old woman who is alert but had a grand mal seizure 2 days ago	Complete	Partial	Shower
A 46-year-old patient who had a motor vehicle accident yesterday, had a mild concussion but no fractures	Complete	Partial	Shower

1-10 INFECTION CONTROL/TRANSMISSION OF ORGANISMS

Provide examples of the following elements found in the **chain of infection:**

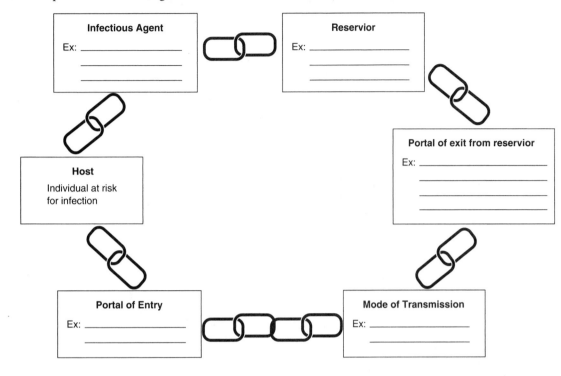

CLINICAL SITUATION   A young woman has recently begun nursing school. During her second week in the clinical setting, she takes care of a 79-year-old client who was admitted with dehydration. The client has a recent history of shingles and is in the convalescent stage of illness. The client's skin is very dry, his oral temperature is 100.4° F. His urine is dark amber and his WBC is 13,000/mm^3.

Pertinent Terminology	Definition
Shingles	
Dehydration	
Incubation Stage	
Prodromal Stage	
Illness Stage	
Convalescent Stage	
Asepsis	
Nosocomial	
Iatrogenic	

From the clinical situation, identify the **factors** that make the client susceptible for getting an infection.

Explain **why** each of the **factors** identified makes the client susceptible to getting an infection.

1. _____

2. _____

3. _____

4. _____

Define **medical asepsis:** _____

_____

Define **surgical asepsis:** _____

_____

In caring for the client, the nurse will use _____ asepsis.

Integrated Learning Activity: With a partner, fill in the diagrams with the proper elements in the chain of infection as it applies to each situation:

1. A family member who has a cold stops in to visit Mr. Wu.

2. A nursing assistant goes from patient to patient without changing gloves.

APPLYING CRITICAL THINKING SKILLS TO TEST QUESTIONS

INSTRUCTIONS: Circle the best answer(s) for each test question. Write your rationale for selecting the answer(s). To enhance your learning and test-taking skills, discuss your answer(s) and rationale(s) with a partner. The answer and the rationale can be found on the back of this page.

1. The nurse is taking care of a client who has a respiratory infection with a productive cough. To promote infection control, the nurse is most correct to (select all that apply):
   a. use alcohol-based hand rubs.
   b. push oral fluids every shift.
   c. have the client use a tissue when coughing.
   d. auscultate the lung sounds every 4 hours.
   e. handwash with non-antimicrobial soap and water.

   Rationale for your selection: _____
   _____
   _____
   _____
   _____
   _____

2. The client has been diagnosed with a gastrointestinal bacteria obtained from drinking contaminated water. In the chain of infection, the water is the:
   a. portal of entry.
   b. reservoir.
   c. portal of exit.
   d. infectious agent.

   Rationale for your selection: _____
   _____
   _____
   _____
   _____
   _____

3. The client's abdominal dressing is described as having a moderate amount of serosanguineous drainage and a very foul odor. In planning the dressing change, it is most important for the nurse to:
   a. apply extra dressings to the wound.
   b. use sterile gloves to change the dressing.
   c. wash her hands before and after the dressing change.
   d. change the abdominal dressing more often.

   Rationale for your selection: _____
   _____
   _____
   _____
   _____
   _____

ANSWER KEY FOR
APPLYING CRITICAL THINKING SKILLS TO TEST QUESTIONS

HELPFUL HINTS: Read all test questions carefully. Identify **key words** in the question that will guide you in answering the question. In these test questions the key words to consider are **"most correct,"** and **"most important."** Compare your rationale with the one in the test question.

1. The nurse is taking care of a client who has a respiratory infection with a productive cough. To promote infection control, the nurse is most correct to (select all that apply):
   a. use alcohol-based hand rubs.
   b. push oral fluids every shift.
   c. have the client use a tissue when coughing.
   d. auscultate the lung sounds every 4 hours.
   e. handwash with non-antimicrobial soap and water.

   Rationale: The answers (a), (c), and (e) are infection control principles and practices recommended by the Centers for Disease Control and Prevention to help reduce the transmission of diseases. Options (b) and (d) are good nursing interventions but are not effective in reducing the transmission of diseases.

2. The client has been diagnosed with a gastrointestinal bacteria obtained from drinking contaminated water. In the chain of infection, the water is the:
   a. portal of entry.
   b. reservoir.
   c. portal of exit.
   d. infectious agent.

   Rationale: The answer is (b). The water is the reservoir that provided the environment for the infectious agent to reproduce. Options (a), (c), and (d) are part of the chain of infection, but the water is the reservoir.

3. The client's abdominal dressing is described as having a moderate amount of serosanguineous drainage and a very foul odor. In planning the dressing change, it is most important for the nurse to:
   a. apply extra dressings to the wound.
   b. use sterile gloves to change the dressing.
   c. wash her hands before and after the dressing change.
   d. change the abdominal dressing more often.

   Rationale: The answer is (c). Handwashing is the single most effective method in decreasing the spread of pathogens. Option (a) can be done, but it is not the most important option; options (b) and (d) are ordered by the practitioner.

1-11 SKIN INTEGRITY

List the **factors** that increase the **risk** for development of a pressure ulcer:

1. _____
2. _____
3. _____
4. _____
5. _____
6. _____
7. _____
8. _____
9. _____
10. _____
11. _____

Use the diagram to **circle** the areas of the body where **pressure ulcers** are likely to develop on a bedridden patient:

CLINICAL SITUATION   An 88-year-old female client has been admitted to the hospital with a fractured left elbow. She is malnourished and weighs only 90 pounds. She is currently confused and a sitter has been assigned at her bedside. The family reports that the client eats less than 50% of her meals and has difficulty walking. The client is anorexic and her skin is soft and thin. She is incontinent of urine.

Pertinent Terminology	Definition
Pressure Ulcer	_____
Necrosis	_____
Ischemia	_____
Reactive Hyperemia	_____
Blanching	_____
Slough	_____
Eschar	_____
Tunneling	_____
Debridement	_____
Excoriation	_____

BRADEN SCALE FOR PREDICTING PRESSURE SORE RISK

Go online and access the Braden Scale at *http://www.bradenscale.com/images/bradenscale.pdf.* **Select the number** on the scale that best applies to the client's risk for development of pressure ulcers (the **lower the number,** the greater is the risk for the development of pressure ulcers).

- After 2 days of taking care of the client, the nurse made the following documentation on the client's medical record: "Reddened, open, dry circular area on sacrum, approximately 2.5 cm × 2.5 cm. Dr. Stanley notified."
- Use the documentation to check off (✓) the **"stage"** of the client's pressure ulcer from the following **Pressure Ulcer Stages:**

Suspected Deep Tissue Injury ☐ Purple or maroon discolored area; intact skin or blood-filled blister.	**Stage I** ☐ Nonblanchable redness of a localized area; intact skin.
Stage II ☐ Partial-thickness dermis loss. Pink wound bed without slough. May present as an intact or open serum-filled blister.	**Stage III** ☐ Full-thickness tissue loss; subcutaneous fat may be visible, but bone, tendon, or muscle are not exposed. Slough, tunneling, and undermining may be present.
Stage IV ☐ Full-thickness tissue loss with exposed bone, tendon, or muscle. Slough and eschar may be present on some parts of the wound bed. Tunneling and undermining is often present.	**Unstageable** ☐ Full-thickness tissue loss in which the base of the ulcer is covered by slough or eschar.

Source: National Pressure Ulcer Advisory Board at *www.npuap.org.*

⚡ **Integrated Learning Activity:** With a partner, **write in** the **"stage"** of the pressure ulcer for each of the following clinical situations using the **Pressure Ulcer Stages**:

Clinical Situation	Pressure Ulcer Stage
A male client was brought to the hospital. He has an open wound on his left heel that is 2 inches wide and ½ inch deep. It has a foul odor and the heel bone is exposed.	
The nurse measures an irregular open wound on the right hip. The subcutaneous tissue is visible.	

APPLYING CRITICAL THINKING SKILLS TO TEST QUESTIONS

INSTRUCTIONS: Circle the one best answer for each test question. Write your rationale for selecting the answer. To enhance your learning and test-taking skills, discuss your answer and rationale with a partner. The answer and the rationale can be found on the back of this page.

1. The nurse is taking care of a client who has a stage I pressure ulcer on the sacrum. In delegating the care of the client, it is most important for the nurse to:
   a. instruct the nursing assistant to turn the client every 2 hours.
   b. ask the nursing assistant to massage the client's sacrum.
   c. review how to assess the client's sacrum with the nursing assistant.
   d. inform the nursing assistant of the client's pressure ulcer.

   Rationale for your selection: _____
   _____
   _____
   _____
   _____
   _____

2. While reading the admission notes of a client, the nurse notes that the physician has identified eschar on the left heel. Which of the following assessments is most significant of this finding?
   a. A black scab like area on the left heel
   b. A bruised area on the left heel
   c. A stage III pressure ulcer on the left heel
   d. A stage IV pressure ulcer on the left heel

   Rationale for your selection: _____
   _____
   _____
   _____
   _____
   _____

3. On turning a client to the lateral position, the nurse notes a reddened area on the right hip. Further assessment reveals intact skin with blanching at the site. Which of the following is the most appropriate nursing intervention?
   a. Notify the physician.
   b. Document the findings.
   c. Apply a dry sterile dressing.
   d. Document the presence of a stage I pressure ulcer.

   Rationale for your selection: _____
   _____
   _____
   _____
   _____
   _____

ANSWER KEY FOR
APPLYING CRITICAL THINKING SKILLS TO TEST QUESTIONS

HELPFUL HINTS: Read all test questions carefully. Identify key words in the question that will guide you in answering the question. In these test questions the **key words** to consider are **"most important," "most significant,"** and **"most appropriate."** Compare your rationale with the one in the test question.

1. The nurse is taking care of a client who has a stage I pressure ulcer on the sacrum. In delegating the care of the client, it is most important for the nurse to:
   a. instruct the nursing assistant to turn the client every 2 hours.
   b. ask the nursing assistant to massage the client's sacrum.
   c. review how to assess the client's sacrum with the nursing assistant.
   d. inform the nursing assistant of the client's pressure ulcer.

   Rationale: The answer is (a). Instructing the nursing assistant to carry out an intervention that would assist in preventing further skin breakdown is most important. Option (b) could cause more tissue damage; option (c) is not appropriate for a nursing assistant to assess; and option (d) is not client centered and does not provide a specific intervention to assist the client.

2. While reading the admission notes of a client, the nurse notes that the physician has identified eschar on the left heel. Which of the following assessments is most significant of this finding?
   a. A black scab like area on the left heel
   b. A bruised area on the left heel
   c. A stage III pressure ulcer on the left heel
   d. A stage IV pressure ulcer on the left heel

   Rationale: The answer is (a), which describes the appearance of eschar. Eschar must be debrided to "stage" the pressure ulcer. Options (b), (c), and (d) do not describe the finding.

3. On turning a client to the lateral position, the nurse notes a reddened area on the right hip. Further assessment reveals intact skin with blanching at the site. Which of the following is the most appropriate nursing intervention?
   a. Notify the physician.
   b. Document the findings.
   c. Apply a dry sterile dressing.
   d. Document the presence of a stage I pressure ulcer.

   Rationale: The answer is (b). A reddened area with intact skin and blanching indicates circulation to the site. Options (a) and (c) are not necessary at this time. For option (d), the findings do not support the definition of a stage I pressure ulcer.

ONE

1-12 COMMUNICATION

List essential **therapeutic communication techniques** used in a helping relationship:

- _____
- _____
- _____
- _____
- _____

- _____
- _____
- _____
- _____
- _____

Identify **nontherapeutic responses** that block the development of therapeutic communication:

- _____
- _____
- _____
- _____
- _____
- _____

Use the diagrams to identify the factors that influence communication

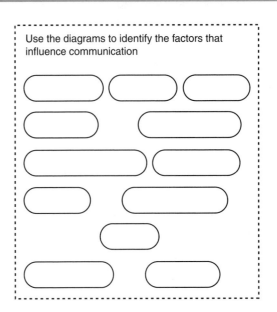

CLINICAL SITUATION Casey, a student nurse, is in the clinical facility for the first time. She is assigned to a 70-year-old female client who was admitted with a fracture of the right hip. The client had her own business for 30 years but is now retired. She remains active in her community. The staff tells the student nurse that the client is a very cranky woman. As soon as Casey walks into the room she hears, "Well, it is about time! If I had to wait any longer I probably would starve to death." Casey responds softly, "I just came on duty."

Pertinent Terminology	Definition
Therapeutic Relationship Orientation Phase	_____
Working Phase	_____
Termination Phase	_____
Paralanguage	_____
Communication	_____

Use the clinical situation to identify **three factors** that would initially affect the development of a therapeutic relationship with the client:

_____   _____   _____

Casey's response to the client is an example of _____.

Casey may have addressed the client's statements by saying: _____
_____

Identify the **therapeutic communication technique** used by Casey in the statement and provide a **rationale** as to why this statement is more appropriate:

Therapeutic Technique	Rationale

 Integrated Learning Activity: With a partner, use the following clinical situations to select the appropriate communication technique or response being used:

(Paraphrasing)   (False reassurance)   (Summarizing)

(Open-ended question)   (Clarification)   (Advising)

1. **Nurse:** "Good morning Mr. S, I heard you had a lot of pain last night. Could you describe the type of pain you had?"

    _____

2. **Family Member:** "The doctor just told me that my husband suffered a severe heart attack!"

    Nurse: "I'm sorry, but don't worry, I'm sure everything will be fine."

    _____

3. **Client:** "I'm just so sick all the time. I just can't do anything by myself anymore. I feel so helpless!"

    Nurse: "It is hard for you to be so dependent and not feel like you are in control. You sound pretty tired of it all."

    _____

4. **Client:** "Nurse, I need to know more information on the pill you gave me this morning."

    Nurse: "Mr. G, I gave you several pills this morning. Which one would you like to know more about?"

    _____

APPLYING CRITICAL THINKING SKILLS TO TEST QUESTIONS

INSTRUCTIONS: Circle the one best answer for each test question. Write your rationale for selecting the answer. To enhance your learning and test-taking skills, discuss your answer and rationale with a partner. The answer and the rationale can be found on the back of this page.

1. The following conversation takes place at the client's bedside:
   Nurse: "Good morning Mr. J, I am your nurse for today. Did you sleep well?"
   Client: "I am not sure."
   Nurse: "You are not sure?"
   Which of the following statements is most accurate of this conversation? The nurse:
   a. should ask a question to validate the client's confusion.
   b. used an appropriate follow-up communication technique.
   c. should look at the chart to see how the client slept.
   d. was inappropriate in asking the second question.

   Rationale for your selection: _____
   _____
   _____
   _____
   _____

2. The nurse walks into a client's room and sees the postsurgical client holding his abdomen and grimacing. The nurse states, "You look like you are in pain." The nurse's statement is:
   a. appropriate because it states what the nurse is observing.
   b. appropriate because pain is expected after surgery.
   c. inappropriate because the nurse made a conclusion before validating.
   d. inappropriate because the nurse should wait for the client to speak first.

   Rationale for your selection: _____
   _____
   _____
   _____
   _____

3. The following conversation takes place at the client's bedside:
   Nurse: "Mr. T, I will be teaching you how to change your surgical dressing."
   Client: "I would prefer that you wait until my wife gets here. She takes care of everything."
   Nurse: "You shouldn't depend on your wife. I'll show you first and then you can teach your wife."
   The nurse's last statement is:
   a. advising the client.
   b. appropriate because it encourages self-care.
   c. having the client reinforce what will be taught.
   d. inappropriate because that nurse should have called the wife first.

   Rationale for your selection: _____
   _____
   _____
   _____
   _____

ANSWER KEY FOR
APPLYING CRITICAL THINKING SKILLS TO TEST QUESTIONS

HELPFUL HINTS: Read all test questions carefully. Identify key words in the question that will guide you in answering the question. In these test questions the **key words** to consider are **"most accurate"** and **"most important."** Compare your rationale with the one in the test question.

1. The following conversation takes place at the client's bedside:
   Nurse: "Good morning Mr. J, I am your nurse for today. Did you sleep well?"
   Client: "I am not sure."
   Nurse: "You are not sure?"
   Which of the following statements is most accurate of this conversation? The nurse:
   a. should ask a question to validate the client's confusion.
   b. used an appropriate follow-up communication technique.
   c. should look at the chart to see how the client slept.
   d. was inappropriate in asking the second question.

   Rationale: The answer is (b). The nurse used a reflective (paraphrase) technique to solicit more information from the client. Options (a), (c), and (d) do not solicit more information.

2. The nurse walks into a client's room and sees the postsurgical client holding his abdomen and grimacing. The nurse states, "You look like you are in pain." The nurse's statement is:
   a. appropriate because it states what the nurse is observing.
   b. appropriate because pain is expected after surgery.
   c. inappropriate because the nurse made a conclusion before validating.
   d. inappropriate because the nurse should wait for the client to speak first.

   Rationale: The answer is (a). The nurse is stating the objective observations. This allows the client to clarify or validate the observation. Options (b), (c), and (d) are not appropriate therapeutic communication techniques that facilitate client communication.

3. The following conversation takes place at the client's bedside:
   Nurse: "Mr. T, I will be teaching you how to change your surgical dressing."
   Client: "I would prefer that you wait until my wife gets here. She takes care of everything."
   Nurse: "You shouldn't depend on your wife. I'll show you first and then you can teach your wife."
   The nurse's last statement is:
   a. advising the client.
   b. appropriate because it encourages self-care.
   c. having the client reinforce what will be taught.
   d. inappropriate because that nurse should have called the wife first.

   Rationale: The answer is (a). The nurse's comment reflects how the nurse feels about the client's decision and does not demonstrate sensitivity to the client. This can cause a block to communication. Options (b), (c), and (d) do not take into consideration the importance of the client's personal needs and social structure.

1-13 REPORTING PATIENT STATUS

List the most common methods nurses use to **report patient status** during the shift and from shift to shift:

1. _____

2. _____

3. _____

4. _____

Place an "X" in the box(es) that best describe(s) the information that should be included in a **handoff report.** The handoff report should:

☐ Provide basic information such as room number, date of admission, and medical diagnosis.

☐ Provide specific information regarding the client's needs and plan of care.

☐ Provide information on significant changes in the client's condition.

☐ Provide information on follow-up client care.

☐ Provide information on clients transferred or discharged from the unit (varies in some hospitals).

CLINICAL SITUATION   0700 (RN, handoff morning report on the following two patients)

"Mr. J in room 461 is a 76-year-old man. He was admitted last night with sepsis. He has an IV of 0.9% normal saline infusing at 75 mL/hr. He is NPO. His output for the shift is 150 mL total. The 0600 temperature is 100.6° F and his blood pressure is 146/94. I am concerned about his temperature and output, so I think it is important to monitor his output and temperature every 4 hours."

"Mr. H in room 462 has been here for 3 days with pneumonia. His temperature at 0600 was 102.4° F and I gave him two Tylenol tablets. His pulse oximetry was 94% on room air. He has an IV infusing at 100 mL/hr and there are 300 mL left. He has a productive cough and is bringing up thick whitish phlegm. I sent the sputum specimen to the laboratory. He has taken in only 50 mL of oral fluid and his output was 275 mL for the shift. I recommend that his temperature be monitored every 2 hours throughout the shift and his intake be discussed with his doctor today."

Pertinent Terminology	Definition
Nursing Rand/Kardex	_____ _____
Worksheet	_____ _____
Reporting	_____ _____
SBAR	_____ _____

Use the **clinical situation** to fill in the worksheet with the pertinent information obtained in morning report on the clients:

Worksheet

| Pt. Name: _____
    Age: _____

VS: _____
_____
Amb. ____ Bed rest ____
Bath (self) ____ (Bed) ____ | Rm: _____

I = _____
O = _____

Diet: _____ | Dx: _____

Admit date _____

IV: _____
_____
_____ | Follow-up Notes:
_____
_____
_____
_____
_____ |
| Pt. Name: _____
    Age: _____

VS: _____
Pulse ox: _____
Amb. ____ Bed rest ____
Bath (self) ____ (Bed) ____ | Rm: _____

I = _____
O = _____

Diet: _____ | Dx: _____

Admit date _____

IV: _____
_____
_____ | Follow-up Notes:
_____
_____
_____
_____
_____
_____ |

Additional information to complete the worksheet is found in the _____

_____ .

⚡ **Integrated Learning Activity:** With a partner, answer the questions regarding (1) the **handoff report** for the following clinical situation, and (2) **fill in the worksheet** and discuss the **follow up notes:**

1500 (**handoff** report)

"Mr. W, 92 years old, in room 357 was admitted yesterday with anemia. His hemoglobin this morning is 7.2 mg/dL and his hematocrit is 26%. He is hard of hearing and weighs 127 pounds. His Foley catheter drained only 100 mL all shift. He has an IV of normal saline solution infusing at 75 mL/hr. He will receive 2 units of blood this evening. The lab will call when the blood is ready. The family and client will make a decision soon regarding his code status. He is very weak and needs a lot of assistance."

• Identify the basic information given in the report: _____

_____

• Identify the significant information given in the report: _____

_____

Worksheet

| Pt. Name: _____
    Age: _____

VS: _____
_____
Amb. ____ Bed rest ____
Bath (self) ____ (Bed) ____ | Rm: _____

I = _____
O = _____

Diet: _____ | Dx: _____

Admit date _____

IV: _____
_____
_____ | Follow-up Notes:
_____
_____
_____
_____ |

1-14 INTRODUCTION TO THE ASSESSMENT PROCESS

List the **methods** available to the nurse for the **collection of patient data:**

1. _____

2. _____

3. _____

4. _____

List the **parts of the patient's medical record** that assist the nurse in the **collection of patient data:**

1. _____

2. _____

3. _____

4. _____

5. _____

6. _____

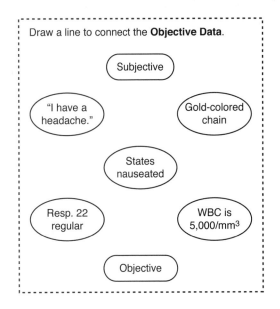

Draw a line to connect the **Objective Data**.

Subjective

"I have a headache."

Gold-colored chain

States nauseated

Resp. 22 regular

WBC is 5,000/mm³

Objective

CLINICAL SITUATION   Mrs. C has been admitted to the hospital for the birth of her baby. Her husband is by her side. You observe that she is very pleasant but cries out with each contraction. She tells you, "I feel a lot of pressure in my back." Her medical record indicates that she is 26 years old and that she has a 6-year-old son.

Pertinent Terminology	Definition
Assessment	_____
Subjective Data	_____
Objective Data	_____
Clustering Data	_____
Validation of Data	_____
Primary Source	_____
Secondary Source	_____

Use the clinical situation to identify the following information:

List the objective data:	Source (Primary/Secondary)
1.	
2.	
3.	
4.	
List the subjective data:	
1.	

Integrated Learning Activity: With a partner, use the box to identify subjective and objective data from the clinical situations:

Mrs. T has been admitted with depression. She answers questions softly with a "yes" or "no" response. She wants her door closed and her room dark. She refuses visitors and eats only 10% of her meals. You notice that she cries regularly and sleeps a lot. She bites her nails frequently.	**Objective Data** **Subjective Data**
Mr. P had surgery 1 day ago. He tells you that he has been very independent all his life and hates being sick. He has refused his pain medication all morning. You notice that he refuses to get out of bed, he moans quietly every now and then, he is sweaty, and his hands are clenched tightly. His surgical dressing is clean and he says everything is fine when you ask him a question.	**Objective Data** **Subjective Data**
Mr. K informs the certified nursing assistant that he is nauseated. He has refused his lunch. You go in to check him and you notice 100 mL of clear yellow emesis. He tells you that he vomited. His wife is at his bedside.	**Objective Data** **Subjective Data**

1-15 BASIC PHYSICAL ASSESSMENT

List the **four methods of examination** used in the performance of a physical assessment:

1. _____

2. _____

3. _____

4. _____

Write in the most appropriate **method(s) of examination** for each of the following:

• Oral mucous membranes

_____

• Peripheral pulses

_____

• Arterial blood pressure

_____

• Lung sounds

_____

• Lower extremity edema

_____

• Apical pulse

_____

• Distended abdomen

_____

CLINICAL SITUATION Carrie is a nursing student assigned to Ms. W. Ms. W, 18 years old, came to the emergency department with complaints of right lower abdominal pain. She was admitted and had an appendectomy the day of admission. She is 1 day postop and will be going home this afternoon. Carrie performs a **body systems assessment** and documents the following notes:

Neuro: Alert and oriented × 4. **Cardiovascular:** Radial pulse regular and bounding. **Skin:** Warm and dry, pallor present, turgor elastic. **Respirations:** Regular, clear. **Gastrointestinal:** Bowel sounds present in all four quadrants. RLQ abdominal dressing clean, complains of tenderness with light palpation. **Genitourinary:** States voiding without difficulty. **Musculoskeletal:** Ambulates with a steady gait. **Psychosocial:** Cheerful.

Pertinent Terminology	Definition
Inspection	_____
Palpation	_____
Percussion	_____
Auscultation	_____
Chief Complaint	_____
Review of Systems	_____

Use the documentation notes from the clinical situation to **identify the method of examination** used by Carrie in performing the body systems assessment:

Documentation	Method(s) of Examination
Neuro: Alert and oriented × 4	
Cardiovascular: Radial pulse regular and bounding	
Skin: Warm and dry, pallor, turgor elastic	
Respirations: Regular, clear	
Gastrointestinal: Bowel sounds present in all four quadrants. Right lower quadrant abdominal dressing clean; complains of tenderness with light palpation	
Genitourinary: States voiding without difficulty	
Musculoskeletal: Ambulates with a steady gait	
Psychosocial: Cheerful	

Integrated Learning Activity: With a partner, use the following documentation notes to identify (1) the body system being assessed, and (2) the method of examination used:

Documentation Notes	Body System Method(s) of Examination
States it is 1945, does not know where he is; knows first name; hand grip strength unequal: right hand grip stronger than left	
Voided 50 mL of amber fluid; abdomen distended	
Warm, moist; pallor with erythema on sacral area; edema 1+ on bilateral lower extremities	
Absent bowel sounds in lower and upper right quadrants, hyperactive on upper and lower left quadrant; having small amounts of liquid dark brown stools	
Wheezes audible on inspiration, coughing, expectorating thick yellowish phlegm	
Apical pulse 116, rapid, irregular; radial pulse 98, rapid, thready, irregular	
Passive range of motion to right hand. Unable to extend and flex fingers	
Left facial drooping; left arm and leg flaccid	

APPLYING CRITICAL THINKING SKILLS TO TEST QUESTIONS

INSTRUCTIONS: Circle the one best answer for each test question. Write your rationale for selecting the answer. To enhance your learning and test-taking skills, discuss your answer and rationale with a partner. The answer and the rationale can be found on the back of this page.

1. The nurse is preparing to assess the neurologic status of an adult client who had a hip fracture 5 days ago and was reported to have been confused during the previous shift. Which statement will provide the nurse with the most appropriate information?
   a. "Can you tell me today's date?"
   b. "Do you know that you are in the hospital?"
   c. "When did you have hip surgery?"
   d. "Tell me where you are right now."

   Rationale for your selection: _____
   _____
   _____
   _____
   _____
   _____

2. The nurse is informed that a newly admitted client is complaining of itching and has a rash all over the body. The most appropriate nursing intervention initially is to:
   a. inform the physician of the objective and subjective complaints.
   b. inspect the client and describe the rash.
   c. ask the client to try not to scratch the areas.
   d. check the medication record for anti-itch medication.

   Rationale for your selection: _____
   _____
   _____
   _____
   _____
   _____

3. The nurse is assigned to a client who was admitted for a blood clot in the right leg. Which of the following describes the appropriate assessment technique initially?
   a. Inspection of the right leg
   b. Light palpation of the right leg
   c. Inspection followed by deep palpation of edematous areas
   d. Light palpation followed by inspection of any reddened areas

   Rationale for your selection: _____
   _____
   _____
   _____
   _____

ANSWER KEY FOR
APPLYING CRITICAL THINKING SKILLS TO TEST QUESTIONS

HELPFUL HINTS: Read all test questions carefully. Identify key words in the question that will guide you in answering the question. In these test questions the **key words** to consider are **"most appropriate"** and **"initially."** Compare your rationale with the one in the test question.

1. The nurse is preparing to assess the neurologic status of an adult client who had a hip fracture 5 days ago and was reported to have been confused during the previous shift. Which statement will provide the nurse with the most appropriate information?
   a. "Can you tell me today's date?"
   b. "Do you know that you are in the hospital?"
   c. "When did you have hip surgery?"
   d. "Tell me where you are right now."

   Rationale: The answer is (d). Eliciting orientation to place is part of assessing client orientation. Options (a) and (b) encourage a "yes" or "no" response, and option (c) may not give accurate data if the client does not remember the date.

2. The nurse is informed that a newly admitted client is complaining of itching and has a rash all over the body. The most appropriate nursing intervention initially is to:
   a. inform the physician of the objective and subjective complaints.
   b. inspect the client and describe the rash.
   c. ask the client to try not to scratch the areas.
   d. check the medication record for anti-itch medication.

   Rationale: The answer is (b). It is most appropriate for the nurse to initially gather data by using the assessment skill of inspection and then to further describe the observations. Options (a), (c), and (d) are follow-up nursing interventions.

3. The nurse is assigned to a client who was admitted for a blood clot in the right leg. Which of the following describes the appropriate assessment technique initially?
   a. Inspection of the right leg
   b. Light palpation of the right leg
   c. Inspection followed by deep palpation of edematous areas
   d. Light palpation followed by inspection of any reddened areas

   Rationale: The answer is (a). Inspection is the initial step in the assessment process that provides information on color, size, shape, and movement of the extremity. Options (b) and (d) are not appropriate initially, and option (c) should not be done in this situation.

1-16 DOCUMENTATION

List the primary documentation (charting) formats used in the clinical settings:

1. _____

2. _____

3. _____

4. _____

5. _____

6. _____

Circle the statements that are **true.**

The patient's medical record is a communication tool.

The RN is legally responsible for the documentation made by student nurses.

Charting entries should be concise.

Flow sheets are not part of the client's chart.

Pertinent Terminology	Definition
APIE Charting	_____ _____
Charting by Exception	_____
Clinical Pathway	_____
Electronic Charting	_____
Narrative Charting	_____
Flow Sheets	_____
Focus Charting	_____
POMR Charting	_____
SOAP Charting	_____ _____

Read and review the charting examples. Identify the charting format for Example #1 and Example #2.

Example #1

Nurses' Notes	
Time	
0800	Alert, oriented ×4. States pain level 5 out of 10, using PCA. Lung sounds clear, unlabored using incentive spirometer. Skin warm, dry. NG to suction draining light brown fluid. BS absent ×4 quads. Abd dressing with 2 cm × 2 cm pinkish drainage. _____ M. Molly RN
0900	Foley discontinued as ordered. _____ M. Molly RN

Charting format: _____

Example #2

ADL Documentation					
Time	0930				
Initials	MM				
Hygiene:					
Bath	Bed		(Assisted)	Self	Shower
Oral care	Self			(Assisted)	
Pericare	(Self)			Cath	
Diet:					
Intake	Brkft		Lunch	Dinner	
%	0				
Fed	Self		Assisted	(NPO)	
Mobility:					
Ambulation	Independent		(Assisted)		
	(Chair)		(BR)		

Charting format: _____

⚡ **Integrated Learning Activity:** With a partner, use the following **Nurses' Notes** to identify five documentation errors. List how these errors should be corrected.

Nurses' Notes	
Time	
0700	Patient sleeping. Resp. 20 regular, unlabored. Skin warm _____ M. Molly RN
0730	Awake, pain level 0. Patient up to bathroom MAEW. c/o dizziness on returning to bed. Pale, assisted back to bed. P 98, irregular. BP 90/60 no c/o pain. Side rails up ×4. _____ M. Molly RN
0830	Patient refused breakfast, c/o mild indegestion. Will check to see what medications are ordered _____ _____ M. Molly RN
0900	Had emesis of 100 mL stated, "Felt better" _____ M. Molly RN

Charting errors:

1. _____
   Correct by: _____

2. _____
   Correct by: _____

3. _____
   Correct by: _____

4. _____
   Correct by: _____

5. _____
   Correct by: _____

1-17 SELF-CONCEPT

List the **four components** of self-concept:

1. _____

2. _____

3. _____

4. _____

For each of the **self-concept** components, **identify two stressors** that affect and contribute to altering the component of:

➤ **Identity** (any two)

_____
_____

➤ **Body image** (any two)

_____
_____
_____

➤ **Self-esteem** (any two)

_____
_____
_____

➤ **Role performance** (any two)

_____
_____
_____

CLINICAL SITUATION   A female client was diagnosed with breast cancer 2 weeks ago and recently had a left mastectomy. She is 32 years old and is married with a 5-year-old daughter. She is very anxious after the surgery and wonders how her husband will react to her. She tells the nurse, "I am so young to have this done." She begins to cry and says that she loves being a mom but doesn't think she can have another child because she would not be able to nurse and care for the baby as she would like to. She is scheduled to begin chemotherapy treatments in 1 week.

Pertinent Terminology	Definition
Self-concept	_____
Identity	_____
Body Image	_____
Self-esteem	_____
Role Performance	_____

Reread the clinical situation and cluster the **objective data** and **subjective data** that relate to the **self-concept** component that is marked with an **"X":**

☐ Identity ☒ Body image ☐ Self-esteem ☐ Role performance	➡ ➡	**Objective data:** **Subjective data:**
☐ Identity ☐ Body image ☐ Self-esteem ☒ Role performance	➡ ➡	**Objective data:** **Subjective data:**

⚡ **Integrated Learning Activity:** With a partner, use the following clinical situation to cluster the objective data and the subjective data related to the **self-concept** component that is marked with an **"X":**

CLINICAL SITUATION   A male client had a heart attack 2 months ago and has lost his job. When he comes to the clinic, his facial expression is tense and he speaks in a hostile voice. During the last visit, he stated: "I can't just sit here, I am the breadwinner of my family." "I'm useless since I had the heart attack!"

☒ Identity ☐ Body image ☐ Self-esteem ☐ Role performance	➡ ➡	**Objective data:** **Subjective data:**
☐ Identity ☐ Body image ☒ Self-esteem ☐ Role performance	➡ ➡	**Objective data:** **Subjective data:**

1-18 CULTURAL ASPECTS OF NURSING

List the **six cultural phenomena** that influence nursing care:

1. _____
2. _____
3. _____
4. _____
5. _____
6. _____

List **two examples** for each of the following:

Communication

_____
_____
_____

Social organizations

_____
_____
_____

Environmental control

_____
_____
_____

Biologic variations

_____
_____
_____

CLINICAL SITUATION   Wendy RN, the home health nurse, visits a 62-year-old Hispanic woman who has had diabetes mellitus for 20 years and currently has a sore on her left foot. The client has missed two of her doctor's appointments and has been soaking her foot in warm salt water every night. The client speaks English but does not like to call the clinic or question the nurse because she does want to bother anyone. She enjoys cooking and eating Mexican food. During the home visit Wendy noticed several religious artifacts and many pictures of the client's children and grandchildren on the wall.

Pertinent Terminology	Definition
Culture	_____ _____
Culture Assessment	_____
Cultural Sensitivity	_____ _____
Cultural Imposition	_____
Assimilation	_____ _____
Ethnocentrism	_____ _____

Use the clinical situation to **identify** the **cultural data** that relate to the **culture phenomena** listed below:

Culture Phenomena	Cultural Data
Communication	
Space	
Time	
Social organization	
Environmental control	
Biological variation	

Integrated Learning Activity: With a partner, use the following clinical situations to (1) underline the pertinent cultural data and (2) identify the possible implications for health care delivery:

Clinical Situation	Health Care Delivery Implication(s)
A Filipino woman is very quiet. She rarely complains and the nurses comment on how she doesn't maintain eye contact when the nurse is speaking.	
A client of Chinese ancestry is 80 years old and requires constant care. She lives with one of her daughters and all the adult family members are involved in caring for her at night.	
Mrs. W has had a miscarriage. She hemorrhaged and her blood count is very low. The physician has recommended a blood transfusion, but Mrs. W refuses because of her religious beliefs.	
An African-American woman comes to the outpatient clinic for blood pressure checks. She tells the nurse that her youngest daughter is about to be married. She is concerned because her other daughter has sickle cell anemia.	
A male client had major surgery yesterday. He does not want to get out of bed and has refused all his pain medication. The nurse knows that he is in pain but wants to respect his wishes.	

APPLYING CRITICAL THINKING SKILLS TO TEST QUESTIONS

INSTRUCTIONS: Circle the one best answer for each test question. Write your rationale for selecting the answer. To enhance your learning and test-taking skills, discuss your answer and rationale with a partner. The answer and the rationale can be found on the back of this page.

1. The nurse is preparing to discuss with the alert elderly Hispanic female client the bronchoscopy procedure scheduled the next day. The client tells the nurse that she wants to wait until her family arrives later. Which nursing action is most appropriate?
   a. Provide the information to the client and answer the family's questions later.
   b. Give the client the bronchoscopy procedure information in Spanish.
   c. Tell the client to call you when her family arrives.
   d. Inform the physician.

   Rationale for your selection: _____
   _____
   _____
   _____
   _____
   _____

2. The nurse is taking care of a client who is scheduled for surgery today. The client asks the nurse to read a passage from the Bible to help her prepare herself for surgery. It is most appropriate for the nurse to:
   a. read the Bible passage.
   b. ask if someone on staff is the same religion as the client.
   c. kindly tell the client that nurses cannot get involved in religious issues.
   d. inquire whether the client would prefer that a religious person be called.

   Rationale for your selection: _____
   _____
   _____
   _____
   _____
   _____

3. The nurse is assigned to a client who believes that wearing a copper bracelet will relieve arthritic pain. In providing care for the client, it is most important for the nurse to:
   a. encourage the client to use anti-inflammatory medication.
   b. inform the client that copper bracelets have no proven medical value.
   c. address the pathophysiologic mechanisms associated with arthritis with the client.
   d. respect the beliefs associated with the copper bracelet by the client.

   Rationale for your selection: _____
   _____
   _____
   _____
   _____
   _____

ANSWER KEY FOR
APPLYING CRITICAL THINKING SKILLS TO TEST QUESTIONS

HELPFUL HINTS: Read all test questions carefully. Identify key words in the question that will guide you in answering the question. In these test questions the **key words** to consider are **"most appropriate"** and **"most important."** Compare your rationale with the one in the test question.

1. The nurse is preparing to discuss with the alert elderly Hispanic female client the bronchoscopy procedure scheduled the next day. The client tells the nurse that she wants to wait until her family arrives later. Which nursing action is most appropriate?
   a. Provide the information to the client and answer the family's questions later.
   b. Give the client the bronchoscopy procedure information in Spanish.
   c. Tell the client to call you when her family arrives.
   d. Inform the physician.

   Rationale: The answer is (c). The family is an important social organization in many cultures. Being available when the family arrives is manifesting respect for the client's wishes and cultural sensitivity. Options (a) and (d) do not address cultural sensitivity. Option (b), although this action demonstrated cultural sensitivity, this initial action assumes the client wants the information in Spanish. It would be preferable to ask the client if she would like the information in English or Spanish.

2. The nurse is taking care of a client who is scheduled for surgery today. The client asks the nurse to read a passage from the Bible to help her prepare herself for surgery. It is most appropriate for the nurse to:
   a. read the Bible passage.
   b. ask if someone on staff is the same religion as the client.
   c. kindly tell the client that nurses cannot get involved in religious issues.
   d. inquire whether the client would prefer that a religious person be called.

   Rationale: The answer is (a). Recognizing the spiritual needs of a client is viewing the client as a whole person with spiritual as well as physical needs. Options (b), (c), and (d) defer the needs of the patient to someone else.

3. The nurse is assigned to a client who believes that wearing a copper bracelet will relieve arthritic pain. In providing care for the client, it is most important for the nurse to:
   a. encourage the client to use anti-inflammatory medication.
   b. inform the client that copper bracelets have no proven medical value.
   c. address the pathophysiologic mechanisms associated with arthritis with the client.
   d. respect the beliefs associated with the copper bracelet by the client.

   Rationale: The answer is (d). Cultural beliefs play an important role in the healing process. This cultural belief does not interfere with the client's well-being. Options (a), (b), and (c) tend to minimize the client's belief.

1-19 DEVELOPING CULTURALLY COMPETENT CARE

List **factors** that **increase cultural awareness:**

1. _____

_____

2. _____

_____

The **Health Care Culture Compass** identifies relevant human experiences and cultural needs encountered in the health care setting. Nurses need to develop an awareness of their own cultural beliefs and values in order to provide culturally competent care.

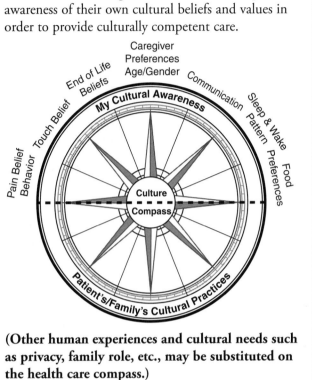

(**Other human experiences and cultural needs such as privacy, family role, etc., may be substituted on the health care compass.**)

CLINICAL SITUATION   The nurse is assigned to Mrs. C, a 45-year-old female patient, who was in a motor vehicle accident. The medical history indicates that Mrs. C is from another country, and she was traveling alone on vacation. She has terminal lung cancer. The patient is conscious but in very critical condition. Per her request, a do-not-resuscitate (DNR) order is written. Her only son will arrive in 3 days.

Pertinent Terminology	Definition
Cultural Awareness	_____ _____
Cultural Competence	_____ _____
Culturally Competent Care	_____ _____
Patient-Centered Care	_____ _____

Use the **healthcare compass** to:

(1) Think about **your own cultural views and beliefs** related to the cultural area identified
by the arrow. Then, fill in the answer below.

Healthcare Compass

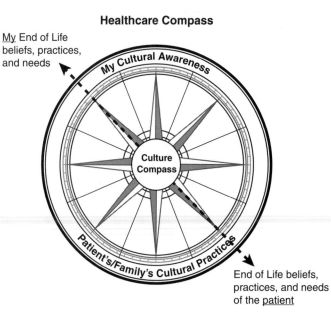

My End of Life
beliefs, practices,
and needs

My Cultural Awareness

Culture
Compass

Patient's/Family's Cultural Practices

End of Life beliefs,
practices, and needs
of the patient

<u>Your own</u> end of life beliefs:

• Spiritual/religious beliefs and practices related to end-of-life care: _____
  _____

Integrated Learning Activity: With a partner, use the clinical situation of Mrs. C to:

• Identify questions that provide the nurse with **knowledge** of Mrs. C's end-of-life cultural beliefs and needs.
  _____
  _____
  _____
  _____

• Identify nursing interventions that reflect **patient-centered culturally competent care.**
  _____
  _____
  _____
  _____

• As Mrs. C is becoming progressively weaker. She whispers to the nurse that her greatest fear is "dying alone."
  Identify nursing interventions that would comfort Mrs. C during this time.
  _____
  _____
  _____
  _____

1-20 INTRODUCTION TO FORMULATING A NURSING DIAGNOSIS

List the **five steps of the nursing process:**

1. _____
2. _____
3. _____
4. _____
5. _____

The **NANDA-I nursing diagnoses** are classified and formulated to address the client's health problems or needs, which can be:

1. _____
2. _____
3. _____
4. _____
5. _____

Use a nursing diagnosis book to write the NANDA-I definition for the following Nursing Diagnoses.

Nursing Diagnosis	NANDA-I Definition
Ineffective Breathing pattern -	_____
Impaired gas exchange -	_____
Acute pain -	_____
Risk for infection -	_____

CLINICAL SITUATION The home health nurse makes the following observations and documents the assessment findings after visiting a 68-year-old male client: Lives alone; his only son lives 60 miles away, visits monthly, and calls weekly. The client stays indoors all day. His vision is poor and he is not able to drive.

Pertinent Terminology	Definition
NANDA-I	_____
Nursing Process	_____
Assessment	_____
Nursing Diagnosis	_____
Defining Characteristics	_____
Planning	_____
Implementation	_____
Evaluation	_____
Related Factors	_____

From the clinical situation, **check off (✓) the nursing diagnosis** most appropriate for the client (use a nursing diagnosis book to validate your selection):

Nursing Diagnoses: ___ Ineffective coping
                         ___ Risk for loneliness
                         ___ Social isolation

List the <u>risk factors</u> or defining characteristics for the nursing diagnosis you selected:

_____   _____   _____

_____   _____

Further documentation by the home health nurse states: The client has lost 10 pounds since the last visit 2 weeks ago. He now demonstrates signs of being malnourished. He lives on a limited income. Needs the services of a nutritionist and a local community service that delivers meals to homebound individuals.

From the **further documentation data, check off (✓) the nursing diagnosis** most appropriate for the client:

Nursing Diagnoses: ___ Social isolation
                         ___ Deficient knowledge
                         ___ Imbalanced nutrition: less than body requirements

List the **current pertinent defining characteristics** for the nursing diagnosis you selected:

_____   _____   _____

⚡ **Integrated Learning Activity:** With a partner, review the following clinical situations and **identify** the **defining characteristics** that relate to the **nursing diagnosis** written next to each situation.

Clinical Situation	Defining Characteristics
The client has a stage II pressure ulcer on her right heel. She has been on bed rest and her right leg is elevated.	IMPAIRED SKIN INTEGRITY _____
The client has oral lesions in his mouth 1 week after receiving chemotherapy. He complains of pain and his mouth is red.	IMPAIRED ORAL MUCOUS MEMBRANES _____
The client is scheduled for surgery in the morning. She says that she is very scared because her grandmother died during surgery.	FEAR _____

1-21 FORMULATING A NURSING DIAGNOSIS

List the components of the:

One-part nursing diagnosis statement:

1. _____

Two-part nursing diagnosis statement:

1. _____

2. _____

Three-part nursing diagnosis statement:

1. _____

2. _____

3. _____

Place an "X" in the box that identifies the common errors made in the development of the nursing diagnosis statement:

☐ Using the NANDA-I diagnostic categories to identify the nursing diagnosis

☐ Using the medical diagnosis in the formulation of the nursing diagnosis

☐ Clustering the subjective/objective data

☐ Using signs and symptoms to write the nursing diagnosis statement

☐ Stating the expected outcome and the diagnostic statement

☐ Using subjective and objective data to identify the nursing diagnosis

☐ Being specific in defining the etiology part of the statement

☐ Stating the medical diagnosis as the etiology

CLINICAL SITUATION   The client is to be scheduled for elective surgery. In preparation for the surgery, the office nurse takes the client's health history. The nurse documents that the client has recently been diagnosed with diabetes mellitus and was prescribed an antidiabetic pill to take every morning. The client tells the nurse that she stopped the "pill" 1 week ago because she was feeling better.

Pertinent Terminology	Definition
Actual Nursing Diagnosis	_____ _____ _____
Risk Nursing Diagnosis	_____ _____
Risk Factors	_____ _____ _____
Etiology	_____ _____ _____
Data Cluster	_____ _____ _____

Use the **clinical situation** to **cluster the subjective** and **objective data.**

Objective data: _____
_____

Subjective data: _____

Use the data to complete the nursing diagnosis below with a **three-part statement** for the client:

Deficient knowledge: _____
_____

✐ **Integrated Learning Activity:** With a partner, review the following clinical situations and (1) list the defining characteristics, (2) identify the error in the nursing diagnosis statement, and (3) write a correct nursing diagnosis:

CLINICAL SITUATION

Throughout the morning, the client has become progressively more confused. He is restless and attempted to get out of bed. He says it is "1982." His laboratory diagnostic studies indicate that he has a decreased serum sodium level. The nurse wrote the following nursing diagnosis:

Chronic confusion, r/t electrolyte imbalance

Defining Characteristics
_____
_____

Error(s)
_____
_____
_____
_____
_____

Nursing Diagnosis
_____
_____
_____
_____

The client goes weekly to the outpatient clinic to have his blood pressure checked. He smokes one pack of cigarettes per day. His blood pressure is 146/88. His father died from heart disease at age 49 years, and his brother is recovering from a heart attack. The nurse writes the following nursing diagnosis:

Risk for heart attack r/t smoking and family history of heart disease

Related Factors
_____
_____
_____
_____

Error(s)
_____
_____
_____
_____

Nursing Diagnosis
_____
_____
_____
_____

APPLYING CRITICAL THINKING SKILLS TO TEST QUESTIONS

INSTRUCTIONS: Circle the one best answer for each test question. Write your rationale for selecting the answer. To enhance your learning and test-taking skills, discuss your answer and rationale with a partner. The answer and the rationale can be found on the back of this page.

1. The nurse clusters the client's objective and subjective signs and symptoms primarily to:
   a. identify the nursing diagnosis.
   b. correlate with the medical diagnosis.
   c. validate the subjective complaints.
   d. work with "risk for" diagnoses.

   Rationale for your selection: _____
   _____
   _____
   _____
   _____
   _____

2. The following nursing diagnosis is found on the client Kardex: Hip fracture r/t fall. In evaluating the written nursing diagnosis, the nurse correctly concludes that the nursing diagnosis:
   a. is written inappropriately.
   b. should be a "risk for" nursing diagnosis.
   c. needs to be written as a three-part statement.
   d. needs the word "acute" in the first part of the statement.

   Rationale for your selection: _____
   _____
   _____
   _____
   _____
   _____

3. The nurse admits an elderly client with the medical diagnosis of dehydration. In developing the nursing diagnoses, it is most important for the nurse to:
   a. establish nursing diagnoses that are based on the medical diagnosis.
   b. focus on nursing diagnoses that affect fluid balance.
   c. gather data to support actual nursing diagnoses.
   d. include actual and "risk for" diagnoses.

   Rationale for your selection: _____
   _____
   _____
   _____
   _____
   _____

ANSWER KEY FOR
APPLYING CRITICAL THINKING SKILLS TO TEST QUESTIONS

HELPFUL HINTS: Read all test questions carefully. Identify key words in the question that will guide you in answering the question. In these test questions the **key words** to consider are **"primarily," "correctly concludes,"** and **"most important."** Compare your rationale with the one in the test question.

1. The nurse clusters the client's objective and subjective signs and symptoms primarily to:
   a. identify the nursing diagnosis.
   b. correlate with the medical diagnosis.
   c. validate the subjective complaints.
   d. work with "risk for" diagnoses.

   Rationale: The answer is (a). Clustering the data helps the nurse to identify the defining characteristic that led to the formulation of a nursing diagnosis. Options (b) and (c) do not apply, and option (d) addresses only "risk for" diagnoses.

2. The following nursing diagnosis is found on the client Kardex: Hip fracture r/t fall. In evaluating the written nursing diagnosis, the nurse correctly concludes that the nursing diagnosis:
   a. is written inappropriately.
   b. should be a "risk for" nursing diagnosis.
   c. needs to be written as a three-part statement.
   d. needs the word "acute" in the first part of the statement.

   Rationale: The answer is (a). Hip fracture is a medical diagnosis. The nurse needs to identify the defining characteristics and then select the appropriate nursing diagnosis. Option (b) is not applicable because hip fracture is an actual client problem, and (c) and (d) do not apply to this example.

3. The nurse admits an elderly client with the medical diagnosis of dehydration. In developing the nursing diagnoses, it is most important for the nurse to:
   a. establish nursing diagnoses that are based on the medical diagnosis.
   b. focus on nursing diagnoses that affect fluid balance.
   c. gather data to support actual nursing diagnoses.
   d. include actual and "risk for" diagnoses.

   Rationale: The answer is (d). Nursing includes the development of actual nursing diagnoses and any "risk for" diagnoses to provide total, safe care to the client. Option (a) is not correct, and options (b) and (c) do not include the monitoring of possible complications.

1-22 ASSESSMENT OF THE ELDERLY PATIENT

List the **interventions** that would assist in communicating with an elderly patient who has hearing loss related to the aging process:

1. _____
2. _____
3. _____
4. _____
5. _____
6. _____

List the **interventions** that would assist an elderly patient who has vision problems related to the aging process:

1. _____
2. _____
3. _____
4. _____
5. _____
6. _____

Mark an **"X"** in the appropriate column that identifies the effects of aging on the following:

	Decreased	Increased
Sensory perception	☐	☐
Visual acuity	☐	☐
Gag reflex	☐	☐
Skin tissue elasticity	☐	☐
Body temperature	☐	☐
Cardiac output	☐	☐
RBC production	☐	☐
Plasma viscosity	☐	☐
Lung capacity	☐	☐
Residual urine	☐	☐

CLINICAL SITUATION   The following information has been given to a group of students regarding the assessment of an elderly patient: Responds slowly but appropriately to all questions. Skin warm, dry, thin, and flaky. Skin turgor greater than 3 sec. Capillary refill greater than 3 sec. Respirations short and shallow, lung sounds with bilateral crackles. 50% intake, states food is very bland. BM this morning moderate amount formed hard stool. Bilateral lower extremities with 1+ pitting edema. Toenails yellowish, thick. Vital signs T 99° F, P 84, R 16, BP 160/80.

Pertinent Terminology	Definition
Arcus Senilis	_____
Edema	_____
Pitting Edema	_____
Kyphosis	_____
Presbycusis	_____
Presbyopia	_____
Turgor	_____

Use the information from the clinical situation to mark an **"X"** on the data that are representative of the normal effects of the aging process:

____ Responds slowly, but appropriately to all questions

____ Skin warm, dry, thin, and flaky

____ Skin turgor greater than 3 sec; capillary refill greater than 3 sec

____ Respirations short and shallow, lung sounds with bilateral crackles

____ 50% intake, states food is very bland

____ BM this morning formed hard stool

____ Bilateral lower extremities with 1+ pitting edema

____ Toenails yellowish, thick

____ Vital signs T 99° F, P 84, R 16, BP 160/80

Integrated Learning Activity: With a partner, use the information provided to **(1) underline** the assessment data that represent the **effects of the normal aging process,** and **(2) select** the NANDA-I nursing diagnosis most appropriate for the situation:

Assessment Data	Nursing Diagnosis
Wife in to see patient, states that husband is confused this morning, does not know that he is in the hospital. Further patient assessment, PERRL, whitish ring noted around the margins of the iris, uses glasses. Mouth dry, wears upper dentures.	☐ Disturbed body image ☐ Impaired oral mucous membrane ☐ Acute confusion ☐ Impaired memory
Skin pale, translucent. Lower extremities thin, pedal pulses weak, palpable. States has loss of a small amount of urine when coughs. Shortness of breath, R 28, mouth breathing. Abdomen round, soft, nontender. Temp. 96.8° F.	☐ Functional urinary incontinence ☐ Hypothermia ☐ Ineffective peripheral tissue perfusion ☐ Ineffective breathing pattern
Transfers independently out of bed, complained of dizziness when coming to a standing position, gait slow. Anterior-posterior diameter of chest increased. Soft diet, intake 70%.	☐ Impaired physical mobility ☐ Risk for injury ☐ Ineffective health maintenance ☐ Imbalanced nutrition: less than body requirements

1-23 CARING FOR THE SURGICAL PATIENT

List the **major** types of anesthesia:

1. _____

2. _____

3. _____

List the **types of regional anesthesia:**

1. _____

2. _____

3. _____

4. _____

5. _____

Identify in which of the perioperative phases **(preoperative, intraoperative, postoperative)** the following interventions would be started:

	Pre	Intra	Post
Use of incentive spirometer	☐	☐	☐
Coughing and deep breathing	☐	☐	☐
Splinting of surgical site	☐	☐	☐
Prepping surgical site	☐	☐	☐
Changing the surgical dressing	☐	☐	☐
Leg exercises	☐	☐	☐
Pain management	☐	☐	☐
Discharge instructions	☐	☐	☐

CLINICAL SITUATION   A female patient is admitted for a total abdominal hysterectomy this morning. She is 52 years old and obese. Her medical history indicates that she stopped smoking 5 years ago. Both parents are deceased. Mother died at the age of 88 years and father died from a heart attack at the age of 62 years. The client's vital signs are T 97.8° F, P 76, R 18, BP 164/92, pain level 0. The following laboratory studies were done: CBC, PT, serum electrolytes of Na^+, K^+, serum FBG, BUN, and creatinine. The UA, chest x-ray report, and ECG report are in the chart.

Pertinent Terminology	Definition
General Anesthesia	_____
Regional Anesthesia	_____
Conscious Sedation	_____
Thrombophlebitis	_____
Atelectasis	_____
Paralytic Ileus	_____
PCA	_____
Sequential Stockings	_____

From the clinical situation, **list** the factors that increase the patient's risk for postoperative complications:

_____   _____
_____   _____

⚡ **Integrated Learning Activity:** With a partner, use the follow-up clinical situation to (1) **identify** which medical order the nurse would do **first** and (2) list the **priority nursing interventions** the nurse would **independently** perform and provide a rationale for each intervention:

FOLLOW-UP CLINICAL SITUATION   The patient returns from the postanesthesia room sleepy but easily arousable. The physician writes the following postoperative orders:

NPO, May have sips of water in the AM
IV: Dextrose 5/0.9% normal saline infuse at 100 mL/hr
Ambulate this evening
VS q30 min for first hour, then q1h ×2 hr, then q4h
Incentive spirometer q1h while awake
PCA with morphine sulfate set at 1 mg/6 min (per patient demand not to exceed 30 mg/4 hr)
Antiembolic stockings and sequential stockings to legs continuously
Indwelling urinary catheter to gravity; remove in AM

First Medical Orders to Implement	Rationale
1.	
Priority Independent Nursing Interventions	**Rationale**
1.	
2.	
3.	
4.	
5.	
6.	
7.	

APPLYING CRITICAL THINKING SKILLS TO TEST QUESTIONS

INSTRUCTIONS: Circle the one best answer for each test question. Write your rationale for selecting the answer. To enhance your learning and test-taking skills, discuss your answer and rationale with a partner. The answer and the rationale can be found on the back of this page.

1. The client is transferred to the surgical unit from the postanesthesia room after having abdominal surgery. There is a J-P drainage device in place. Which of the following reported findings on transfer requires immediate follow-up?
   a. Abdominal dressing reinforced in the recovery room
   b. R 14, P 86, BP 126/90, lethargic but responds to touch
   c. Bowel sounds absent in all quadrants
   d. J-P compressed with 10 mL reddish drainage

   Rationale for your selection: _____
   _____
   _____
   _____
   _____

2. Which of the following client statements is correct in describing the appropriate use of the incentive spirometer?
   a. "I will first inhale then blow into the mouthpiece."
   b. "I will put the mouthpiece in my mouth and blow into the mouthpiece."
   c. "I will put the mouthpiece in my mouth and then inhale slowly."
   d. "I will put the mouthpiece in my mouth, inhale, and hold for 5 seconds."

   Rationale for your selection: _____
   _____
   _____
   _____
   _____

3. The nurse is preparing a client for emergency surgery. Before surgery, it is most important for the nurse to ensure that the:
   a. preop checklist is completed.
   b. preop medications are documented.
   c. lab results are in the medical record.
   d. surgical consent is signed.

   Rationale for your selection: _____
   _____
   _____
   _____
   _____

ANSWER KEY FOR
APPLYING CRITICAL THINKING SKILLS TO TEST QUESTIONS

HELPFUL HINTS: Read all test questions carefully. Identify key words in the question that will guide you in answering the question. In these test questions the **key words** to consider are **"immediate," "correct,"** and **"most important."** Compare your rationale with the one in the test question.

1. The client is transferred to the surgical unit from the postanesthesia room after having abdominal surgery. There is a J-P drainage device in place. Which of the following reported findings on transfer requires immediate follow-up?
   a. Abdominal dressing reinforced in the recovery room
   b. R 14, P 86, BP 126/90, lethargic but responds to touch
   c. Bowel sounds absent in all quadrants
   d. J-P compressed with 10 mL reddish drainage

   Rationale: The answer is (a). Reinforcement of the surgical dressing indicates excessive drainage; this should be carefully monitored. Option (b) indicates vital signs within normal limits, and options (c) and (d) are expected findings for a client who had abdominal surgery.

2. Which of the following client statements is correct in describing the appropriate use of the incentive spirometer?
   a. "I will first inhale then blow into the mouthpiece."
   b. "I will put the mouthpiece in my mouth and blow into the mouthpiece."
   c. "I will put the mouthpiece in my mouth and then inhale slowly."
   d. "I will put the mouthpiece in my mouth, inhale, and hold for 5 seconds."

   Rationale: The answer is (c). This describes the procedure appropriately. Options (a) and (b) do not describe the procedure correctly, and option (d) is partially correct but the client does not need to hold for 5 seconds.

3. The nurse is preparing a client for emergency surgery. Before surgery, it is most important for the nurse to ensure that the:
   a. preop checklist is completed.
   b. preop medications are documented.
   c. lab results are in the medical record.
   d. surgical consent is signed.

   Rationale: The answer is (d). Although the physician is responsible for obtaining the client's signature, it is most important for the nurse to ensure that it has been signed. Options (a), (b), and (c) are important but are not the most important.

1-24 WOUND ASSESSMENT

List the **types of wounds:**

1. _____

2. _____

List the **types of wound drainage** systems:

1. _____

2. _____

3. _____

4. _____

Match the **wound classifications and wound drainage terminology** with the appropriate description or characteristics:

1. Laceration
2. Contusion
3. Penetrating
4. Abrasion
5. Incision
6. Serosanguineous
7. Serous
8. Sanguineous
9. Purulent

_____ Thin, clear, watery secretion
_____ Containing pus
_____ Open cut made with a knife/scalpel
_____ Containing RBCs
_____ Irregular wound tear; jagged edges
_____ Entering into the tissues/body cavity
_____ Closed wound; with pain, swelling, and discoloration
_____ Red, watery secretion
_____ A scraping away of the skin surface

CLINICAL SITUATION Mr. J, 26 years old, received a stab wound to his abdomen and was taken to the emergency department. He underwent emergency surgery. He has an IV, nasogastric tube to continuous low wall suction, and one Jackson-Pratt on the right upper quadrant and another on the left lower quadrant of the abdomen. He has a closed abdominal wound and the dressing is clean and dry as he is taken to the surgical unit at 0800.

Pertinent Terminology	Definition
Primary Intention	_____
Secondary Intention	_____
Tertiary Intention	_____
Granulation Tissue	_____
Inflammatory Phase	_____
Proliferation Phase	_____
Maturation Phase	_____
Dehiscence	_____
Evisceration	_____

Use the clinical situation to **check off** (✔) all the factors that apply to Mr. J:

☐ High risk for infection   ☐ Postop pain should initially increase

☐ Healing by secondary intention   ☐ J-P drainage should progressively decrease

☐ J-P will aid in the healing process   ☐ Slight redness around incision first day

Three hours after arriving on the surgical unit, the nurse took the vital signs and noted that Mr. J's surgical dressing has two abd pads and the dressing is currently saturated with sanguineous drainage. The nurse lightly palpated the abdomen.

Implement the appropriate nursing interventions on the abdominal surgical dressing:

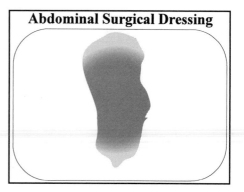

Abdominal Surgical Dressing

Select the nurse's documentation that demonstrates appropriate assessment:

____ Abdominal dressing with large amount of red drainage, abdomen tender, T 100.4° F

____ Abdominal dressing covered with pink reddish drainage, abdomen tender, no bowel sounds, P 88, BP 136/86

____ Abdominal dressing saturated with red drainage, abdomen tender, reinforced, P 88, BP 136/86

⚡ **Integrated Learning Activity:** With a partner, use the statements below to (1) check (✔) whether the statement is correct or incorrect and (2) provide a rationale for your selection.

Statements	Correct/Incorrect	Rationale
1. Wound drainage devices need to be emptied once a shift.	☐ Correct ☐ Incorrect	
2. Wound drainage devices need to be compressed to function.	☐ Correct ☐ Incorrect	
3. Assessment of the wound should be done once a day.	☐ Correct ☐ Incorrect	
4. Wound description does not need to include wound measurement.	☐ Correct ☐ Incorrect	
5. Wound evisceration requires the application of sterile dry gauze.	☐ Correct ☐ Incorrect	

APPLYING CRITICAL THINKING SKILLS TO TEST QUESTIONS

INSTRUCTIONS: Circle the one best answer for each test question. Write your rationale for selecting the answer. To enhance your learning and test-taking skills, discuss your answer and rationale with a partner. The answer and the rationale can be found on the back of this page.

1. An elderly client is being discharged after abdominal surgery. The staples were removed on the third day after surgery and a gauze dressing was applied. The client tells the nurse that as he was standing up he heard a pop coming from his abdomen. Which nursing intervention is of priority?
   a. Fully assess the neurologic status of the client.
   b. Auscultate the bowel sounds.
   c. Assess the surgical site.
   d. Palpate the abdomen.

   Rationale for your selection: _____
   _____
   _____
   _____
   _____
   _____

2. On the second day after surgery, the nurse assesses a surgical wound and documents the following, "Surgical incision with stitches intact, erythema noted on surrounding skin around surgical incision, edges well approximated." On the basis of this documentation, the nurse most accurately assessed that the surgical wound:
   a. is healing without complications.
   b. is beginning to show signs of complications.
   c. needs to be assessed by the physician.
   d. will take longer to heal.

   Rationale for your selection: _____
   _____
   _____
   _____
   _____
   _____

3. The physician orders the following dressing changes for an elderly client who has an open wound on the sacrum: "Apply hydrocolloid dressing on the wound. Change dressing every 3 days." A primary purpose of this dressing is to:
   a. enhance healing by primary intention.
   b. decrease the need for daily dressing changes.
   c. protect the wound from additional pressure.
   d. maintain a moist wound environment.

   Rationale for your selection: _____
   _____
   _____
   _____
   _____
   _____

ANSWER KEY FOR
APPLYING CRITICAL THINKING SKILLS TO TEST QUESTIONS

HELPFUL HINTS: Read all test questions carefully. Identify key words in the question that will guide you in answering the question. In these test questions the **key words** to consider are **"priority," "most accurately,"** and **"primary purpose."** Compare your rationale with the one found for each question.

1. An elderly client is being discharged after abdominal surgery. The staples were removed on the third day after surgery and a gauze dressing was applied. The client tells the nurse that as he was standing up he heard a pop coming from his abdomen. Which nursing intervention is of priority?
   a. Fully assess the neurologic status of the client.
   b. Auscultate the bowel sounds.
   c. Assess the surgical site.
   d. Palpate the abdomen.

   Rationale: The answer is (c). Wound dehiscence is a possible complication. Clients may not have any pain. With option (a) not enough data are present to suggest that a full neurologic assessment is warranted, and options (b) and (d) should be done after inspection.

2. On the second day after surgery, the nurse assesses a surgical wound and documents the following, "Surgical incision with stitches intact, erythema noted on surrounding skin around surgical incision, edges well approximated." On the basis of this documentation, the nurse most accurately assessed that the surgical wound:
   a. is healing without complications.
   b. is beginning to show signs of complications.
   c. needs to be assessed by the physician.
   d. will take longer to heal.

   Rationale: The answer is (a). Documentation describes the normal healing process of a second post-operative day surgical wound. Options (b), (c), and (d) are not appropriate at this time.

3. The physician orders the following dressing changes for an elderly client who has an open wound on the sacrum: "Apply hydrocolloid dressing on the wound. Change dressing every 3 days." A primary purpose of this dressing is to:
   a. enhance healing by primary intention.
   b. decrease the need for daily dressing changes.
   c. protect the wound from additional pressure.
   d. maintain a moist wound environment.

   Rationale: The answer is (d). Hydrocolloid dressings help to remove exudates from a wound and maintain a moist environment to promote healing. Option (a) is incorrect because the wound will heal by secondary intention; options (b) and (c) are not the primary purpose for applying this dressing.

ONE

1-25 WOUND DRESSINGS

List the **types of wound dressings:**

1. _____

2. _____

3. _____

4. _____

5. _____

Alginate: _____
_____

Hydrogel: _____
_____

Hydrocolloid: _____
_____

Transparent: _____
_____

Wet-dry gauze dressing: _____
_____
_____

CLINICAL SITUATION   Mr. Y, 78 years old, has been in the acute care setting for 2 months. He was admitted with a fractured left hip, anorexia, and weight loss. He has a stage IV pressure ulcer on the sacrum with undermining at 12 o'clock and a stage II pressure ulcer of the right heel. The physician writes the following orders: irrigate the sacral wound daily with normal saline solution. Pack wound with a wet-dry dressing with normal saline solution every shift. Apply a hydrocolloid dressing to the right heel every 3 days.

Pertinent Terminology	Definition
Debridement	_____
Exudate	_____
Macerate	_____
Mechanical Debridement	_____
Wound Irrigation	_____
Wet-Dry	_____

The nurse is preparing to irrigate and change the dressing of the sacral wound. Select all the statements that apply to the wound irrigation and to the application of the wet-dry dressing.

Wound Irrigation	Sacral Wet-Dry Dressing
☐ Clean the wound bed with iodine	☐ Lightly pack the moist gauze into the wound bed
☐ Use a 35-mL syringe	☐ Pack the dry dressing into the wound first
☐ Irrigate with 0.9% normal saline solution	☐ Lightly pack the area of undermining with the moist dressing
☐ Use a 3-mL syringe with a 22-gauge needle	☐ Lightly pack the area of undermining with the dry dressing
☐ Attach an 18-gauge angiocath to the irrigating syringe	☐ Allow the moist dressing to cover the irrigating syringe outside surface of the skin

---

The nurse writes the following data on the clinical worksheet:

Sacral wound
0900 Size 3.5 cm by 4.0 cm, irregular margins. Pressure ulcer 2.5 cm deep. Slough at margins. Tan-colored drainage moderate amount. Checked for undermining. 1.2 cm undermining at 12 o'clock. Old dressing removed. Wet-dry dressing applied. Irrigated with saline solution with a large syringe. Medicated with analgesic 30 minutes before procedure. Tolerated well.

Right heel wound
0900 Hydrocolloid dressing changed on right heel. No changes from the previous dressing change 3 days ago.

Integrated Learning Activity: With a partner, discuss the wound assessment observations made by the nurse. For the **sacral wound,** rewrite the assessment observations in the space provided.

For the **right heel wound,** identify why the documentation made by the nurse is *not* appropriate.

1-26 THE PATIENT WITH FLUID AND ELECTROLYTE IMBALANCE

List the **adult normal values** for the following electrolytes:

1. Sodium (Na^+) = _____

2. Potassium (K^+) = _____

3. Chloride (Cl^-) = _____

4. Calcium (Ca^{++}) = _____

5. Phosphate (PO_4^{-3}) = _____

6. Magnesium (Mg^{++}) = _____

Write in the appropriate medical terminology for the serum laboratory values below:

Mg^{++} 3.5 mg/dL   = _____

K^+ 2.5 mEq/L   = _____

Cl^- 90 mEq/L   = _____

Na^+ 132 mEq/L   = _____

Ca^{++} 8.5 mg/dL   = _____

PO_4^{-3} 5.1 mg/dL = _____

CLINICAL SITUATION   A 36-year-old client was admitted with gastroenteritis. He has been vomiting and having severe diarrhea for 2 days. He is very weak. The current laboratory results are Na^+ 128 mEq/L, K^+ 2.8 mEq/L, and Cl^- 90 mEq/L. The physician orders an IV of 0.9% normal saline solution with 20 mEq KCL at 100 mL/hr, NPO, and I & O.

Pertinent Terminology	Definition
Sodium (Na^+)	
Potassium (K^+)	
Chloride (Cl^-)	
Calcium (Ca^{++})	
Phosphate (PO_4^{-3})	
Magnesium (Mg^{++})	
Third Space	
Edema	
Pitting Edema	

From the clinical situation, identify the abnormal laboratory results. List the **major clinical signs or symptoms** that you would assess with each abnormal value:

_____	=	_____

_____ = _____

_____ = _____

FOLLOW-UP CLINICAL SITUATION The client's vomiting and diarrhea has begun to subside in the evening, and the MD has ordered a clear liquid diet. The client's **24-hour I & O** for the day is charted below:

24-Hour Intake/Output Record

IV	=	2400	Emesis	=	950
Oral	=	120	Diarrhea	=	900
			Urine	=	750
		2520 mL			**2600 mL**

On the basis of the clinical situation and intake and output record, **select** the most appropriate **NANDA-I nursing diagnoses** for the client:

___ Excess fluid volume   ___ Deficient fluid volume

___ Diarrhea   ___ Impaired skin integrity

___ Imbalanced nutrition: less than   ___ Risk for injury
      body requirements

Integrated Learning Activity: With a partner, read the following clinical situation and write a rationale for each of the nursing interventions listed:

Clinical Situation	Nursing Interventions	Rationale
Ms. M was admitted with heart failure. The nursing diagnosis of "Fluid volume excess r/t noncompliance to dietary Na^+ restriction" is listed in her NCP. Digoxin 0.25 mg qAM po, furosemide 40 mg qAM po, and K-Dur 10 mEq po tid are her medications.	Weigh daily	
	Monitor I & O	
	Take apical pulse	
	Assess skin	
	Assess lungs	
	Assess for peripheral edema	
	✓ Neck veins	

1-27 ELIMINATION—URINARY

List the **factors** that affect bladder elimination:

1. _____

2. _____

3. _____

4. _____

5. _____

6. _____

7. _____

8. _____

9. _____

Use the diagrams to **select** the appropriate size of the indwelling catheter for the female and male patient. **Draw a line** on the catheter at the anticipated length of insertion.

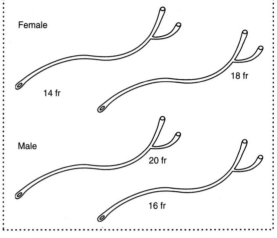

Female

14 fr

18 fr

Male

20 fr

16 fr

CLINICAL SITUATION   Mrs. S, a 42-year-old woman, had abdominal surgery 2 days ago. She has an IV infusing into her left forearm, an indwelling urinary catheter (Foley), and she has a temperature of 100.4° F this evening. She states her pain level is about 2 out of 10. The physician orders the indwelling catheter to be removed in the AM.

Pertinent Terminology	Definition
UA	
Nocturia	
Hematuria	
Dysuria	
Oliguria	
Anuria	
Urinary Incontinence	
Residual Urine	
Midstream UA	
Void	
Indwelling Catheter	
Condom Catheter	

Using the information in the clinical situation, the nurse gathers more information and documents on Mrs. S's chart. **Select the statement** below that describes a thorough observation of the urinary system:

1. Indwelling catheter patent to gravity, taking fluids liberally

2. Indwelling catheter to gravity, draining cloudy, pale yellow urine

3. Indwelling catheter patent to gravity, output 75 mL

4. Indwelling catheter patent, draining freely; abdomen without distention

> The next morning, the nurse prepares to remove the indwelling catheter. Identify the equipment the nurse needs to gather to properly remove the catheter.
>
> _____
>
> The indwelling catheter is removed at 0800. The nurse knows that Mrs. S should void within _____ hours after removal of the catheter.

Integrated Learning Activity: With a partner, **select the NANDA-I nursing diagnosis** that is most appropriate to the clinical situations below that describe the complications Mrs. S had after removal of the indwelling catheter.

NANDA-I nursing diagnoses: (1) Stress urinary incontinence   (2) Urinary retention
                               (3) Impaired urinary elimination   (4) Risk for infection

Clinical Situation	Nursing Diagnosis
Mrs. S is unable to void 8 hours after removal of the indwelling catheter. She has abdominal discomfort, a sensation of fullness, and frequent dribbling.	
Mrs. S is catheterized for residual urine and 700 mL of urine are drained from the bladder. An indwelling catheter is left in place again.	
The following day the catheter is removed. Mrs. S is able to void without any further problems that day. The next day she complains of dysuria when she voids.	
Mrs. S is started on an antibiotic. She notices that the dysuria and hematuria are no longer present. However, she tells you that she has a history of losing urine when she coughs or sneezes.	

APPLYING CRITICAL THINKING SKILLS TO TEST QUESTIONS

INSTRUCTIONS: Circle the one best answer for each test question. Write your rationale for selecting the answer. To enhance your learning and test-taking skills, discuss your answer and rationale with a partner. The answer and the rationale can be found on the back of this page.

1. The physician writes the following order on admission for an adult female patient, "Insert Foley catheter stat." It is most appropriate for the nurse to initially insert a:
   a. 14 F catheter.
   b. 16 F catheter.
   c. 20 F catheter.
   d. 22 F catheter.

   Rationale for your selection: _____
   _____
   _____
   _____
   _____
   _____

2. The nurse is caring for a client who has a urinary catheter. To accurately assess the urine color, it is most important for the nurse to:
   a. look at the color and amount of urine in the drainage bag.
   b. draw 1 to 2 mL of urine from the catheter port.
   c. look at the color of the urine in the drainage tube.
   d. review the color of the urine documented by the previous shift.

   Rationale for your selection: _____
   _____
   _____
   _____
   _____
   _____

3. The physician writes the following order: "I & O cath for residual this AM." Which statement, given to a nursing assistant by the nurse, is most helpful for implementing this order?
   a. "Let me know when the client wants to void."
   b. "Let me know as soon as the client voids."
   c. "Push fluids this morning."
   d. "Record how much the client voids this morning."

   Rationale for your selection: _____
   _____
   _____
   _____
   _____
   _____

ANSWER KEY FOR
APPLYING CRITICAL THINKING SKILLS TO TEST QUESTIONS

HELPFUL HINTS: Read all test questions carefully. Identify key words in the question that will guide you in answering the question. In these test questions the **key words** to consider are **"most appropriate," "accurately assess," "most important,"** and **"most helpful."** Compare your rationale with the one in the test question.

1. The physician writes the following order on admission for an adult female patient, "Insert Foley catheter stat." It is most appropriate for the nurse to initially insert a:
   a. 14 F catheter.
   b. 16 F catheter.
   c. 20 F catheter.
   d. 22 F catheter.

   Rationale: The answer is (a). The nurse will insert the smallest catheter to avoid trauma and unnecessary dilation of the urethra. Option (b) can be used if a 14 F catheter is not available. Options (c) and (d) are too large in diameter for a routine catheterization.

2. The nurse is caring for a client who has a urinary catheter. To accurately assess the urine color, it is most important for the nurse to:
   a. look at the color and amount of urine in the drainage bag.
   b. draw 1 to 2 mL of urine from the catheter port.
   c. look at the color of the urine in the drainage tube.
   d. review the color of the urine documented by the previous shift.

   Rationale: The answer is (c). The color of the urine is best noted in the drainage tube because the tube contains the most recent urine coming from the bladder. Option (b) is used to obtain a urine specimen, option (a) is not the best because urine collecting in the bag may look darker, and option (d) does not provide the most current assessment of the urine.

3. The physician writes the following order: "I & O cath for residual this AM." Which statement, given to a nursing assistant by the nurse, is most helpful for implementing this order?
   a. "Let me know when the client wants to void."
   b. "Let me know as soon as the client voids."
   c. "Push fluids this morning."
   d. "Record how much the client voids this morning."

   Rationale: The answer is (b). Catheterizing for residual requires that the procedure be implemented as soon as the client voids. This will provide information as to the amount of urine left in the bladder after the client has voided. Options (a), (c), and (d) do not address the directions needed for implementing the order.

1-28 ELIMINATION—BOWEL

List the **factors** that affect bowel elimination:

1. _____

2. _____

3. _____

4. _____

5. _____

6. _____

7. _____

Use the diagram to identify the location and placement of the stethoscope when listening for bowel sounds. Draw a **circle** at each location.

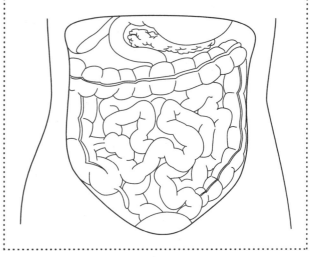

CLINICAL SITUATION   The physician writes the following on the history and physical form after examining a 55-year-old client, Mr. M: Complains of cramping abdominal pain, borborygmi, 5-6 dark brown semi-liquid BMs per day for several days. Last bowel movement this AM. Indicates no changes in diet intake. Denies melena, constipation, nausea, or vomiting. The MD orders an endoscopy, barium enema, and stool for occult blood.

Pertinent Terminology	Definition
Bowel Sounds	_____ _____
Flatus	_____ _____
Constipation	_____ _____
Diarrhea	_____ _____
Occult Blood	_____ _____
Melena	_____ _____
Enema	_____ _____
Fecal Impaction	_____ _____
Borborygmi	_____ _____
Endoscopy	_____ _____
Barium Enema	_____ _____

Using the information identified in the history and physical, identify the questions that the nurse could ask Mr. M to **assess** the bowel pattern changes that he is currently experiencing:

1. Complains of cramping abdominal pain, borborygmi

   Question: _____

2. 5-6 dark brown semiliquid BMs per day for several days

   Question: _____

3. Indicates no changes in diet intake

   Question: _____

4. Denies melena, constipation, nausea, or vomiting

   Question: _____

5. Last bowel movement this AM

   Question: _____

Write two questions that would be useful in further assessing Mr. M's bowel function:

1. _____

2. _____

Discuss how these questions contribute to the assessment.

⚡ **Integrated Learning Activity:** With a partner, select the **NANDA-I nursing diagnosis** that best applies to each of the case clinical situations below:

NANDA-I nursing diagnoses: (1) Perceived constipation   (2) Diarrhea
                             (3) Constipation   (4) Bowel incontinence

Clinical Situation	Nursing Diagnosis
The client takes a mild laxative every night since his retirement 1 year ago. He believes that his change in activity will cause him bowel problems.	
The client was in a car accident 1 month ago in which she sustained a neuromuscular back injury. While hospitalized she was having involuntary frequent loose BMs.	
The nursing diagnosis for Mr. M in the clinical situation is:	

ONE

1-29 GENERAL NUTRITION

List the **four basic diets** commonly encountered in the clinical setting (exclude the special diets):

1. _____

2. _____

3. _____

4. _____

List the most common methods of providing enteral nutrition:

1. _____

2. _____

3. _____

Draw a line to connect the following **foods** with the appropriate **common therapeutic diets** encountered in the clinical setting.

Clear Liquid

Ice cream
Carbonated beverages
Broth fat-free
Cooked vegetables
Cream of rice
Soft   Puddings
Smooth peanut butter
Clear fruit juices
Bananas
Custard
Sherbert
Eggs

Full Liquid

CLINICAL SITUATION   A 68-year-old male client had a cerebral vascular accident 2 weeks ago. He has right-sided hemiplegia. The nursing care rand indicates that the client is on a soft pureed diet with thickened liquids and is on intake and output.

Pertinent Terminology	Definition
Regular Diet	
Soft Diet	
Full Liquid	
Clear Liquid	
Pureed	
Enteral Nutrition	
Gastric Gavage	
Nasogastric Tube	
PEG	
Jejunostomy Tube	

Use the information from the clinical situation to **mark an "X"** on the most appropriate feeding guidelines for the client who has right-sided hemiplegia:

Feeding Guidelines

☐ Give water frequently with the food
☐ Check right cheek for "pocketing"
☐ Place in semi-Fowler position
☐ Teach and allow family to feed Mr. G

☐ Place in high Fowler position
☐ Give thickened juices
☐ Provide oral care
☐ Lie flat after feeding

Integrated Learning Activity: With a partner, use the clinical situations related to the client. For each situation, **prioritize the NANDA-I nursing diagnosis. #1** = Priority, **#2** = Important, and **#3** = Need to monitor.

Clinical Situation	NANDA-I Nursing Diagnosis
The client's intake for last 24 hr = 1250 mL and his output = 725 mL. He is fatigued and needs to be reminded to drink and eat. His skin is dry and flaky. Skin turgor—tenting. Oral mucous membranes dry, several teeth missing. Urine color is dark yellow.	__ Deficient fluid volume r/t decreased fluid intake secondary to fatigue __ Risk for impaired oral mucous membranes r/t insufficient intake of fluids __ Risk for impaired skin integrity r/t dry, thin skin secondary to aging
The client began to cough forcefully while being fed. The feeding was stopped and the MD ordered for him to be NPO. The client has lost 3 pounds in 1 week. He has an IV of D5W infusing at 75 mL/hr. It is difficult to get him out of bed because he is weak and does not assist with the transfer.	__ Imbalanced nutrition: less than body requirements r/t inability to ingest food __ Risk for aspiration r/t impaired swallowing __ Risk for impaired skin integrity r/t prolonged bed rest

1-30 GASTROINTESTINAL TRACT

List the structures in the gastrointestinal tract involved with the digestion and absorption of food:

1. _____

2. _____

3. _____

4. _____

Use the diagram to **identify the quadrants** (RLQ, RUQ, LLQ, LUQ) and the **anatomical regions of the abdomen** (Right and Left Lumbar, Right and Left Inguinal, Umbilical, Epigastric, Suprapubic, and Right and Left Hypochondriac)

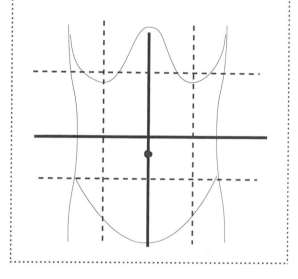

Modified from Black JM, Hawks JH, Keene AM: *Medical-surgical nursing: clinical management for positive outcomes*, ed 8, St. Louis, 2009, WB Saunders.

CLINICAL SITUATION   Mrs. T is a 55-year-old woman who was admitted to the hospital with complaints of diarrhea for the past 10 days. She states that she has abdominal cramping and at times passes bloody stools. She is scheduled for a colonoscopy at 10:00 AM today.

Pertinent Terminology	Definition
Duodenum	
Jejunum	
Ileum	
Cecum	
Colon	
Rectum	
Polyp	

Use the clinical situation to **check off (✓) all the nursing interventions and physician's orders** that you would associate with the preparation of Mrs. T for the colonoscopy procedure.

☐ NPO for procedure

☐ GoLytely will be given for stool evacuation

☐ Monitor for abdominal pain and bleeding after the procedure

☐ Consent is necessary

☐ May have a clear liquid breakfast

☐ Requires general anesthesia

Match the gastrointestinal diagnostic tests with the appropriate definitions:

Diagnostic Test		Definition
1. Colonscopy	__	Visualization of the rectum and sigmoid
2. Endoscopy	__	Visualization from anus to cecum
3. Sigmoidoscopy	__	Visualization of esophagus, stomach, and small bowel
4. Barium swallow	__	Visualization of interior organs and structures using a fiberoptic instrument

Integrated Learning Activity: With a partner, use the diagram to:

1. Identify the segments of the large intestine.
2. Follow the path of the colonoscopy procedure.
3. Identify the consistency of the stool as it moves through the intestinal tract (mushy, semiliquid, and solid).

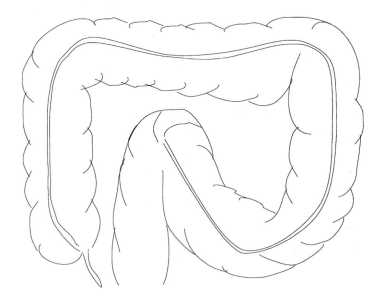

APPLYING CRITICAL THINKING SKILLS TO TEST QUESTIONS

INSTRUCTIONS: Circle the one best answer for each test question. Write your rationale for selecting the answer. To enhance your learning and test-taking skills, discuss your answer and rationale with a partner. The answer and the rationale can be found on the back of this page.

1. The client is scheduled for an UGI endoscopy. Which statement is correct in providing the client with information about this endoscopic procedure?
   a. "A tube will be passed from your nose into your stomach."
   b. "The tube is small, is very flexible, and has a light at the end."
   c. "The tube has a light that will allow the doctor to see your intestines."
   d. "A tube will be passed from your mouth and into your stomach."

   Rationale for your selection: _____
   _____
   _____
   _____
   _____
   _____

2. The day after having a barium enema as an outpatient, the client calls the clinic nurse to express concern because the stools are white in color. Which statement made by the nurse is most helpful?
   a. "Don't worry; this is normal after a barium enema."
   b. "This is expected; be sure to drink plenty of fluids."
   c. "The stool color should return after 1 to 2 days."
   d. "This is expected; call back if your stools are still white after 5 days."

   Rationale for your selection: _____
   _____
   _____
   _____
   _____
   _____

3. The nurse is taking care of a 76-year-old client who is having an upper GI series this morning. After the completion of the procedure, the nurse should initially:
   a. see whether a laxative is ordered for the client.
   b. assess the bowel sounds.
   c. take the vital signs.
   d. observe for intestinal obstruction.

   Rationale for your selection: _____
   _____
   _____
   _____
   _____
   _____

ANSWER KEY FOR
APPLYING CRITICAL THINKING SKILLS TO TEST QUESTIONS

HELPFUL HINTS: Read all test questions carefully. Identify key words in the question that will guide you in answering the question. In these test questions the **key words** to consider are **"correct,"** **"most helpful,"** and **"initially."** Compare your rationale with the one in the test question.

1. The client is scheduled for an UGI endoscopy. Which statement is correct in providing the client with information about this endoscopic procedure?
   a. "A tube will be passed from your nose into your stomach."
   b. "The tube is small, is very flexible, and has a light at the end."
   c. "The tube has a light that will allow the doctor to see your intestines."
   d. "A tube will be passed from your mouth and into your stomach."

   Rationale: The answer is (d). This is a beginning statement that informs the client as to how the procedure will be carried out. Options (a), (b), and (c) do not provide accurate information about the procedure.

2. The day after having a barium enema as an outpatient, the client calls the clinic nurse to express concern because the stools are white in color. Which statement made by the nurse is most helpful?
   a. "Don't worry; this is normal after a barium enema."
   b. "This is expected; be sure to drink plenty of fluids."
   c. "The stool color should return after 1 to 2 days."
   d. "This is expected; call back if your stools are still white after 5 days."

   Rationale: The answer is (b). It is important to reassure the client and to provide instructions that help minimize complications. Barium impaction is a concern after a barium enema. Options (a), (c), and (d) do not provide enough information.

3. The nurse is taking care of a 76-year-old client who is having an upper GI series this morning. After the completion of the procedure, the nurse should initially:
   a. see whether a laxative is ordered for the client.
   b. assess the bowel sounds.
   c. take the vital signs.
   d. observe for intestinal obstruction.

   Rationale: The answer is (a). To prevent the complication of fecal impaction after an UGI series (barium swallow), a laxative is usually given after the procedure. Options (b) and (c) are good interventions, but the situation does not address the need for these interventions; option (d) does not focus on the initial intervention.

1-31 DIABETES MELLITUS

List the classic **symptoms** of **diabetes mellitus:**

1. _____
2. _____
3. _____

List other **signs** and **symptoms** associated with **hyperglycemia:**

1. _____
2. _____
3. _____
4. _____
5. _____
6. _____
7. _____

Fill in the circles that identify the signs and symptoms associated with **hypoglycemia.**

O Polyuria   O Shakiness

O Tremor

O Behavior changes   O Glucosuria

O Polydipsia

O Sweating   O Confusion

O Dizziness   O Headache

O Hunger

O Slurred speech

O Paresthesia   O Tachycardia

CLINICAL SITUATION   A 20-year-old woman makes an appointment with her physician for complaints of feeling fatigued and lethargic for several days. She states that she has noticed that she has lost 15 pounds. She tells the physician that she does not understand why she has lost so much weight since she has been eating a lot. The physician asks whether she voids more than usual. The client says that she does but that she thinks it is because of all the water that she is drinking all day.

Pertinent Terminology	Definition
Diabetes Mellitus (DM)	
Type 1 Diabetes	
Type 2 Diabetes	
Insulin Resistance	
Insulin	
Counterregulatory	
Oral Hypoglycemic Agents	
Fasting Plasma Glucose (FPG)	
Casual Blood Glucose	

The client's physician orders a fasting plasma glucose (FPG) test. Another FPG and a 2-hr oral glucose tolerance test (OGTT) are also ordered. The following results are noted in the client's clinic chart. **Write** the normal laboratory value for the test in the column provided.

Test	Results	Normal Laboratory Values
FPG	130 mg/dL	
FPG	160 mg/dL	
OGTT 2-hr postload glucose	225 mg/dL	

The client is informed that she has type 1 diabetes mellitus. **Fill in** the circles that correlate with the diagnosis and treatment of type 1 diabetes mellitus.

O   Oral hypoglycemics will be ordered   O   Will require blood glucose testing

O   Exercise is part of the treatment plan   O   Beta cells are producing insulin

O   Will need to monitor for signs and   O   Will need to monitor for signs and
    symptoms of hyperglycemia   symptoms of hypoglycemia

O   Insulin will be required every day   O   Will not need insulin if follows diet

Integrated Learning Activity: With a partner, match each question in the **follow-up clinical situation** with the appropriate response(s) in the **Key Points Box.** Next to each question, **write** the letter(s) of the responses you have selected.

Key Points Box

A. "Usually 30 min to 1 hr before breakfast."	**E.** "Destroyed by the gastric enzymes."
B. "Insulin needs may change over time."	**F.** "No."
C. "Check blood sugar level."	**G.** "Drink apple or grape juice."
D. "Always carry oral glucose tablets."	**H.** "Know the signs and symptoms of hypoglycemia."

FOLLOW-UP CLINICAL SITUATION   The patient is started on Humulin N insulin 15 units qAM and Humulin N 5 units qPM. She is taught how to do self-monitoring blood glucose checks (SMBG) qid.

Client's Questions	Responses
1. "When is the best time to administer the AM insulin?"	
2. "If I forget the PM dose of insulin, can I double the dose in the morning?"	
3. "What should I do if I begin to get shaky and dizzy?"	
4. "How do I prepare for a hypoglycemic reaction?"	

ONE

APPLYING CRITICAL THINKING SKILLS TO TEST QUESTIONS

INSTRUCTIONS: Circle the one best answer for each test question. Write your rationale for selecting the answer. To enhance your learning and test-taking skills, discuss your answer and rationale with a partner. The answer and the rationale can be found on the back of this page.

1. A client is diagnosed with diabetes mellitus type 1. In teaching the client about diabetes mellitus type 1, it is most important for the client to:
   a. know how to use oral hypoglycemic agents to control the diabetes.
   b. understand that insulin injections will be required daily.
   c. randomly check fingerstick blood glucose throughout the day.
   d. decrease physical activity.

   Rationale for your selection: _____
   _____
   _____
   _____
   _____
   _____

2. The nurse learns in handoff morning report that the 0700 fasting blood glucose of a client was 72 mg/dL. Which of the following morning assessment findings is of priority?
   a. Abdominal wound dressing with moderate dried red drainage.
   b. Complaining of thirst and dried mouth.
   c. Output of 250 mL during the night shift.
   d. Diaphoresis noted while taking vital signs.

   Rationale for your selection: _____
   _____
   _____
   _____
   _____
   _____

3. The nurse is assigned to a client who has just been diagnosed with diabetes mellitus type 1. Which of the following assessment findings is most consistent with this diagnosis?
   a. FPG 110 mg/dL, hypertension, decreased urinary output
   b. Casual blood glucose of 140 mg/dL, obese, limited physical activity
   c. Weight loss, episodes of shakiness and diaphoresis
   d. Frequent urination, hunger, and excessive fluid intake

   Rationale for your selection: _____
   _____
   _____
   _____
   _____
   _____

ANSWER KEY FOR
APPLYING CRITICAL THINKING SKILLS TO TEST QUESTIONS

HELPFUL HINTS: Read all test questions carefully. Identify key words in the question that will guide you in answering the question. In these test questions the **key words** to consider are **"most important," "priority,"** and **"most consistent."** Compare your rationale with the one in the test question.

1. A client is diagnosed with diabetes mellitus type 1. In teaching the client about diabetes mellitus type 1, it is most important for the client to:
   a. know how to use oral hypoglycemic agents to control the diabetes.
   b. understand that insulin injections will be required daily.
   c. randomly check fingerstick blood glucose throughout the day.
   d. decrease physical activity.

   Rationale: The answer is (b). With diabetes mellitus type 1, the beta cells have stopped functioning and the use of exogenous insulin administration is required. Option (a) is not appropriate for type 1 diabetes mellitus because hypoglycemic oral agents are used for type 2 DM. Option (c) is incorrect because blood glucose is monitored at specific times for control; option (d) is incorrect because exercise is recommended.

2. The nurse learns in handoff morning report that the 0700 fasting blood glucose of a client was 72 mg/dL. Which of the following morning assessment findings is of priority?
   a. Abdominal wound dressing with moderate dried red drainage.
   b. Complaining of thirst and dried mouth.
   c. Output of 250 mL during the night shift.
   d. Diaphoresis noted while taking vital signs.

   Rationale: The answer is (d). Diaphoresis is a sign associated with hypoglycemia and should be assessed further. Also, the morning blood glucose was toward the lower limit of normal. Options (a) and (c) are within normal limits, and option (b) is important but not a priority.

3. The nurse is assigned to a client who has just been diagnosed with diabetes mellitus type 1. Which of the following assessment findings is most consistent with this diagnosis?
   a. FPG 110 mg/dL, hypertension, decreased urinary output
   b. Casual blood glucose of 140 mg/dL, obese, limited physical activity
   c. Weight loss, episodes of shakiness and diaphoresis
   d. Frequent urination, hunger, and excessive fluid intake

   Rationale: The answer is (d). The classic signs and symptoms associated with diabetes mellitus type 1 are polyuria, polydipsia, and polyphagia. Options (a), (b), and (c) are not the most consistent with the diagnosis.

1-32 COMPLICATIONS OF DIABETES MELLITUS

List the **causes** that precipitate **hypoglycemic reactions:**

1. _____
2. _____
3. _____
4. _____
5. _____

List the **causes** that precipitate the development of **diabetic ketoacidosis:**

1. _____
2. _____
3. _____

For each line identify a specific **long-term complication,** e.g., stroke, associated with diabetes mellitus.

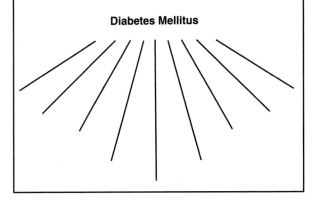

Diabetes Mellitus

CLINICAL SITUATION   Mr. E, 56 years old, has been a diabetic for 25 years. He is admitted to the hospital after having a cerebral vascular accident (CVA). His wife says that her husband monitors his blood glucose daily and administers his own insulin. However, she tells the nurse that he does not always stick to his diet. She wonders whether this may have contributed to the CVA. Mr. E has an order for Humulin N insulin 36 units qAM and Humulin N 12 units qPM with fingerstick blood glucose checks ac and hour of sleep. He is started on a correction bolus insulin scale (sliding scale).

Pertinent Terminology	Definition
Lipoatrophy	_____
	_____
	_____
Lipohypertrophy	_____
	_____
	_____
Impaired Fasting Glucose	_____
	_____
Dawn Phenomenon	_____
	_____
	_____
Diabetic Ketoacidosis (DKA)	_____
	_____
	_____
Hyperglycemic Hyperosmolar Nonketotic Syndrome (HHNS)	_____
	_____

Use the **clinical situation, the follow-up information, and the nursing interventions below** to plan out Mr. E's morning care in the order of **priority.** Place a number, beginning with #1, in each box to indicate the sequence of the nursing care that should be delivered by the nurse.

Follow-up information: The AM blood glucose fingerstick and insulin are to be done by the morning shift. Mr. E is started on a diet containing semithick liquids.

1.— 2.— 3.—	Nursing Interventions	Rationale
	Perform a body systems assessment	
	Perform a fingerstick	
	Take the AM vital signs	
	Administer morning insulin	
	Perform morning care	
	Provide information regarding the complications of diabetes	
	Assist with breakfast	

Place a check (✔) next to the statements that are correct regarding the use of a correction bolus insulin scale (sliding scale).

☐ Regular or rapid-acting insulin is used   ☐ Used for patients with diabetes mellitus type 1

☐ Dosage based on ac blood glucose levels   ☐ Used for patients with diabetes mellitus type 2

☐ May be mixed with all other insulins   ☐ Used during periods of illness

Integrated Learning Activity: The following nursing diagnosis is found on Mr. E's nursing care plan. With a partner, write the three most important nursing interventions for the nursing diagnosis.

Nursing Diagnosis	Nursing Interventions
Risk for aspiration r/t impaired swallowing secondary to CVA	1.
	2.
	3.

APPLYING CRITICAL THINKING SKILLS TO TEST QUESTIONS

INSTRUCTIONS: Circle the one best answer for each test question. Write your rationale for selecting the answer. To enhance your learning and test-taking skills, discuss your answer and rationale with a partner. The answer and the rationale can be found on the back of this page.

1. The nurse notes that the assigned client has an AV fistula on the right arm and is scheduled for hemodialysis this morning. In delegating the care of the client, it is most important for the nurse to:
   a. inform the nursing assistant to give the bath after the hemodialysis.
   b. direct that all morning care is done before hemodialysis.
   c. instruct that the blood pressure be taken on the left arm.
   d. ask that the client be weighed first.

   Rationale for your selection: _____
   _____
   _____
   _____
   _____
   _____

2. The nurse is admitting a client with uncontrolled diabetes mellitus with a history of cerebral vascular accident and left-sided hemiparesis. The client's admitting blood glucose level was 325 mg/dL. Which of the following nursing diagnosis is of priority?
   a. Risk for deficient fluid volume
   b. Deficient fluid volume
   c. Ineffective peripheral tissue perfusion
   d. Noncompliance

   Rationale for your selection: _____
   _____
   _____
   _____
   _____
   _____

3. The nurse is taking care of a client who has diabetes mellitus type 1. The client tells the nurse that he is beginning to feel shaky and experiencing symptoms of hypoglycemia. Which action by the nurse is of priority?
   a. Have the client drink a glass of apple juice.
   b. Monitor for signs of hypoglycemia.
   c. Take the pulse, respirations, and blood pressure.
   d. Have the laboratory perform a blood glucose test stat.

   Rationale for your selection: _____
   _____
   _____
   _____
   _____
   _____

ANSWER KEY FOR
APPLYING CRITICAL THINKING SKILLS TO TEST QUESTIONS

HELPFUL HINTS: Read all test questions carefully. Identify key words in the question that will guide you in answering the question. In these test questions the **key words** to consider are **"most important"** and **"priority."** Compare your rationale with the one in the test question.

1. The nurse notes that the assigned client has an AV fistula on the right arm and is scheduled for hemodialysis this morning. In delegating the care of the client, it is most important for the nurse to:
   a. inform the nursing assistant to give the bath after the hemodialysis.
   b. direct that all morning care is done before hemodialysis.
   c. instruct that the blood pressure be taken on the left arm.
   d. ask that the client be weighed first.

   Rationale: The answer is (c). It is most important to ensure the patency of the AV fistula and prevent vascular complications that can occur with applied pressure from the BP cuff. Options (a) and (b) can be done anytime, and although option (d) is important, it is not the most important on the basis of this situation.

2. The nurse is admitting a client with uncontrolled diabetes mellitus with a history of cerebral vascular accident and left-sided hemiparesis. The client's admitting blood glucose level was 325 mg/dL. Which of the following nursing diagnosis is of priority?
   a. Risk for deficient fluid volume
   b. Deficient fluid volume
   c. Ineffective peripheral tissue perfusion
   d. Noncompliance

   Rationale: The answer is (a). The body will attempt to excrete the excessive glucose and will also excrete water and electrolytes, predisposing the client to dehydration. Options (b), (c), and (d) are important, but they are not priorities during the acute phase.

3. The nurse is taking care of a client who has diabetes mellitus type 1. The client tells the nurse that he is beginning to feel shaky and experiencing symptoms of hypoglycemia. Which action by the nurse is of priority?
   a. Have the client drink a glass of apple juice.
   b. Monitor for signs of hypoglycemia.
   c. Take the pulse, respirations, and blood pressure.
   d. Have the laboratory perform a blood glucose test stat.

   Rationale: The answer is (a). The hypoglycemic effects can occur rapidly. It is always better to treat hypoglycemia in the early stages, before there are signs of central nervous system involvement. Options (b), (c), and (d) do not focus on the immediate treatment.

MEMORIZE generic names

1-33 INSULIN THERAPY

List the **onset, peak,** and **duration** of the following insulins:

Rapid-acting:
  Onset _____ 15 min
  Peak _____ 60-90 min
  Duration _____ 3-4 hrs

Short-acting:
  Onset _____ 1/2 - 1 hour
  Peak _____ 2-3 hours
  Duration _____ 3-6 hours

Intermediate-acting:
  Onset _____ 2-4 hours
  Peak _____ 4-10 hours
  Duration _____ 10-16 hours

Long-acting:
  Onset _____ 1-2 hours
  Peak _____ N/A
  Duration _____ 24 + hours

has to be in own syringe

In the boxes in the left column write **(R)** if the insulin is rapid acting, **(S)** if the insulin is short acting, **(I)** if the insulin is intermediate acting, and **(L)** if the insulin is long acting.

L	Lantus (glargine)	
R	Humalog Mix 50/50	
S	Humulin R	
I	Humulin N	
R	Humalog (lispro)	
R	Novalog (aspart)	
R	Apidra (glulisine)	
L	Levemir (detemir)	

In the boxes on the right side, place an **"X"** to identify the insulin that may be given **IV.**

CLINICAL SITUATION Marty, 22 years old, has been on Humulin N insulin since her diagnosis of type 1 diabetes mellitus 2 years ago. Marty administers 12 units Humulin N with 5 units Humulin R insulin qAM and 4 units Humulin N qPM. She monitors her blood glucose qid AC and hour of sleep and routinely administers the AM insulin dose at 0700 and the PM dose at 1700. Marty maintains a daily chart of her blood glucose results.

before meals

Pertinent Terminology	Definition
Glucagon	
Glycogenolysis	
Gluconeogenesis	
Glycosylated Hemoglobin	
Basil Insulin	
Bolus Insulin	
Hypoglycemia	

From the clinical situation, plot out Marty's morning dose of Humulin N and Humulin R insulin on the **Insulin Progression Graph.** Begin with the **onset (O)** followed by identifying the **peak of action (P)** of the insulin and the **duration (D).**

Insulin Progression Graph
Onset → Peak → Duration

Length of time insulin remains in the body

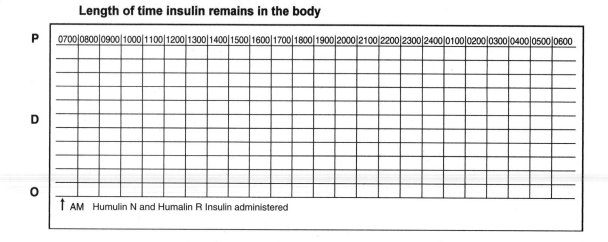

| P | 0700 | 0800 | 0900 | 1000 | 1100 | 1200 | 1300 | 1400 | 1500 | 1600 | 1700 | 1800 | 1900 | 2000 | 2100 | 2200 | 2300 | 2400 | 0100 | 0200 | 0300 | 0400 | 0500 | 0600 |

↑ AM   Humulin N and Humalin R Insulin administered

Marty eats a full breakfast 0800 but is unable to eat lunch. Use the **Insulin Progressive Graph** to indicate the time Marty would most likely experience a **hypoglycemic episode.** ___1200___

Select (✓) the most appropriate **snack** for Marty to eat if she experiences a hypoglycemic reaction at 1600 and has a fingerstick blood glucose of 64 mg/dL

_____ 6 saltine crackers

__X__ 4 oz apple juice

_____ 8 oz diet soda

 Integrated Learning Activity: With a partner, **underline** the **correct word** in each statement as it relates to the sentence and provide a rationale for your selection.

1. For the patient with diabetes mellitus type 1, moderate exercise may have **hyperglycemic** or **hypoglycemic** effects.

   Rationale: _____

   _____

2. A patient with diabetes mellitus type 1 performs a fingerstick before exercising, and the blood glucose results are 92 mg/dL. The patient should eat a snack **before** or **immediately after** exercising.

   Rationale: _____

   _____

3. Excess alcohol consumption puts the patient with diabetes mellitus type 1 at risk for **hypoglycemia** or **hyperglycemia.**

   Rationale: _____

   _____

ONE

APPLYING CRITICAL THINKING SKILLS TO TEST QUESTIONS

INSTRUCTIONS: Circle the one best answer for each test question. Write your rationale for selecting the answer. To enhance your learning and test-taking skills, discuss your answer and rationale with a partner. The answer and the rationale can be found on the back of this page.

1. The nurse learns in report that the assigned client has a fingerstick blood glucose result of 100 mg/dL at 0700. The client receives Humulin N insulin 15 units subcut qAM. On the basis of the morning handoff report, it is most appropriate for the nurse to:
   a. hold the AM dose of insulin.
   b. administer the AM dose of insulin.
   c. call the physician to report the blood glucose results.
   d. repeat the fingerstick blood glucose test at 0800.

   Rationale for your selection: _____
   _____
   _____
   _____
   _____
   _____

2. The physician orders Humulin N insulin 23 units subcut qAM. The nurse carries out this order correctly when the insulin:
   a. dose is given after breakfast.
   b. dose is based on the fingerstick blood glucose results.
   c. is given according to the hospital's qAM schedule.
   d. is administered before breakfast.

   Rationale for your selection: _____
   _____
   _____
   _____
   _____
   _____

3. A client with diabetes mellitus type 1 has a correction bolus insulin scale (sliding scale) with Humulin R insulin listed on the patient care rand. Based on this finding, it is most important for the nurse to:
   a. administer the Humulin R insulin on the basis of the fasting blood glucose level.
   b. monitor the client's urine for ketones before meals.
   c. obtain fingerstick blood glucose test before meals.
   d. check the fingerstick blood glucose qid.

   Rationale for your selection: _____
   _____
   _____
   _____
   _____
   _____

ANSWER KEY FOR
APPLYING CRITICAL THINKING SKILLS TO TEST QUESTIONS

HELPFUL HINTS: Read all test questions carefully. Identify key words in the question that will guide you in answering the question. In these test questions the **key words** to consider are **"most appropriate," "correctly,"** and **"most important."** Compare your rationale with the one in the test question.

1. The nurse learns in report that the assigned client has a fingerstick blood glucose result of 100 mg/dL at 0700. The client receives Humulin N insulin 15 units subcut qAM. On the basis of the morning handoff report, it is most appropriate for the nurse to:
   a. hold the AM dose of insulin.
   b. administer the AM dose of insulin.
   c. call the physician to report the blood glucose results.
   d. repeat the fingerstick blood glucose test at 0800.

   Rationale: The answer is (b). The fingerstick blood glucose results are within normal limits. The nurse should administer the daily dose of insulin. Options (a), (c), and (d) are not appropriate interventions in this situation.

2. The physician orders Humulin N insulin 23 units subcut qAM. The nurse carries out this order correctly when the insulin:
   a. dose is given after breakfast.
   b. dose is based on the fingerstick blood glucose results.
   c. is given according to the hospital's qAM schedule.
   d. is administered before breakfast.

   Rationale: The answer is (d). Although daily insulin is ordered qAM, the ordered dose is given before breakfast to correlate with the action of the insulin and food intake. Options (a) and (c) are similar and start after food intake. Option (b) is used mostly with regular insulin.

3. A client with diabetes mellitus type 1 has a correction bolus insulin scale (sliding scale) with Humulin R insulin listed on the patient care rand. Based on this finding, it is most important for the nurse to:
   a. administer the Humulin R insulin on the basis of the fasting blood glucose level.
   b. monitor the client's urine for ketones before meals.
   c. obtain fingerstick blood glucose test before meals.
   d. check the fingerstick blood glucose qid.

   Rationale: The answer is (c). The correction bolus insulin scale (sliding scale) is used to administer regular insulin throughout the day on the basis of fingerstick blood glucose levels. Options (a), (b), and (d) do not correlate the purpose of the correction bolus insulin scale (sliding scale), regular insulin, blood glucose, and food intake.

1-34 LEGAL CONSIDERATIONS IN NURSING PRACTICE

List the **two types** of **torts:**

1. _____

2. _____

List the **four elements** that constitute **professional negligence:**

1. _____

2. _____

3. _____

4. _____

Draw a line to identify the **Unintentional Torts.**

Fraud   Invasion of privacy

UNINTENTIONAL TORTS

Assault

Negligence

False imprisonment

Libel

Malpractice

CLINICAL SITUATION   Cassie, a new nursing student, is assigned to Mr. W, a 73-year-old client. Mr. W has kidney disease and has been in the hospital for 3 days. He is alert and wants to know everything about his treatment and questions the nurses all the time. The handoff report indicates that he has had diarrhea all day. He keeps getting out of bed, and the nurses feel that he is getting increasingly weak. Cassie is working with an experienced staff RN. The staff RN instructs Cassie to raise all four bedside rails on Mr. W because she is concerned that he will fall and injure himself.

Pertinent Terminology	Definition
Assault	_____
Battery	_____
Libel	_____
Slander	_____
Negligence	_____
Malpractice	_____
Tort	_____
Informed Consent	_____
Standard of Care	_____

Use the information in the clinical situation to **check off (✔)** the statement or statements below that apply to the situation:

☐ A physician's order is not needed since Mr. W is increasingly weak and the nurse has determined that he is a risk to himself.

☐ The patient's behavior is considered unsafe behavior and bedside rails are not considered restraints.

☐ Raising all four bedside rails would potentially be considered a form of restraint.

☐ It is important to follow the instructions of the experienced RN because she alone is responsible for the care that Mr. W receives.

Integrated Learning Activity: With a partner, use the clinical situations below to **(1)** check off **(✔)** the most appropriate action(s) and **(2)** answer the question at the end of the clinical situation.

Clinical Situation	Action(s)
Cindi, a second-year nursing student, has been under a lot of personal stress. She tells another student that she gave her patient the wrong amount of sedative in the morning but that the patient was fine because she carefully monitored his vital signs all day. Cindi is an excellent student and will not allow this to happen again.	☐ The patient was fine—take no action ☐ Fill out an incident/adverse event report ☐ The instructor should be notified ☐ The charge nurse should be notified ☐ The physician should be notified

Cindi **has** or **has not** *(circle one)* been negligent, because _____

_____

Clinical Situation	Action(s)
Mark is a graduate nurse and started working as soon as he received his RN license. He administered medications through the patient's nasogastric tube. During the administration of the medication, the patient began coughing forcefully and gasping for air, Mark noticed that the nasogastric tube had been significantly out of the patient's nose.	☐ Notify the physician ☐ Reinsert tube and listen for placement ☐ Fill out an incident/adverse incident report ☐ Readminister the medications

Mark **has** or **has not** *(circle one)* been negligent, because _____

_____

1-35 REVIEW QUESTIONS

Instructions: Select the most appropriate answer for the following multiple-choice questions.

1. The registered nurse of the medical unit is informed that four clients on the unit have dehydration and diarrhea after eating food contaminated with *Escherichia coli*. Which nursing intervention is most effective in preventing the spread of the organism?
   a. Putting any meat found on the meal tray in the microwave for 2 minutes.
   b. Wearing gloves when bathing clients and assisting the clients.
   c. Assigning one nurse to care for the four clients.
   d. Washing hands frequently when caring for the clients.

2. A mother called the clinic nurse to ask whether her son might get head lice because he used a set of earphones, 2 days ago, that he borrowed from a friend who was just diagnosed with head lice. Which information is most correct information to share with the mother? (Select all that apply.)
   a. It is very unlikely that headphones transmit the head lice.
   b. Head lice need head-to-head contact to spread.
   c. Use a lice shampoo immediately, even if head lice are not visible.
   d. Adult head lice that lay the eggs do not live for more than 24 hours.
   e. Dogs and cats can also transmit head lice.

3. The following vital signs are charted on the adult client's medical record chart for the day shift: 0800, T 98° F, P 88 (regular), R 24, BP 128/88; 1200, T 99.4° F, P 92 (regular), R 22, BP 124/80. After reviewing the medical record, which follow-up nursing intervention is most appropriate for the day shift nurse to implement?
   a. Retake the temperature in 1 hour.
   b. Begin cooling measures.
   c. Maintain the client on bed rest until the temperature is normal.
   d. Contact the physician for an antipyretic medication.

4. The nurse is caring for a client who was admitted 2 days ago with hypertension and atrial tachycardia. The handoff report indicates that the client's pulse at 0600 was 122. To apply the assessment phase of the nursing process, it is most important for the nurse to:
   a. ensure that the pulse has been reported to the physician.
   b. plan to monitor the pulse rate q2h.
   c. review the pulse rates for the last 48 hours.
   d. administer the cardiac medications on time.

5. On auscultating the lung sounds of the assigned client, the nurse hears loud vesicular breaths sounds on the anterior lateral aspects of chest during inspiration. The most appropriate follow-up action by the nurse is to:
   a. have the client use the incentive spirometer q1h while awake.
   b. monitor the client for shortness of breath q2h.
   c. check the client's pulse oximetry.
   d. document the findings.

6. The nurse auscultates the abdominal quadrants of a client and immediately hears soft gurgling bowel sounds. Which action by the nurse is most appropriate?
   a. Reassess the bowel sounds in 15 minutes.
   b. Document the findings as assessed.
   c. Chart the bowel sounds as "borborygmus."
   d. Ask another nurse to assess the bowel sounds.

7. The nurse is assigned to a client who has an indwelling urinary catheter and is placed under contact precautions. The nursing care plan indicates that the client has methicillin-resistant *Staphylococcus aureus* in the urine. To prevent the spread of infection, it is most important for the nurse to:
   a. wear a mask whenever entering the client's room.
   b. wear sterile gloves when coming in contact with the client's urine.
   c. use a gown, gloves, and mask when bathing the client.
   d. use a gown, gloves, and eye protection to empty the client's urinary catheter.

8. The nurse is bathing an elderly client at 0800. On turning the client, the nurse finds a small white tablet on the bed. The client takes Lasix (a small white tablet) at 0700 and 1700. It is most appropriate for the nurse to:
   a. document that a small white tablet was found on the client's bed.
   b. administer another dose of Lasix now.
   c. inform the client that the morning dose of Lasix was found on the bed.
   d. recommend that the medications be mixed with soft food to avoid client noncompliance.

9. An elderly client is telling the nurse the names of his grandchildren who are in a photograph. Suddenly the client begins to cry. Which action is most appropriate initially?
   a. Ask the client why he is crying.
   b. Ask the client if he would like to contact his family.
   c. Tell the client that it is difficult to be sick.
   d. Tell the client that you are sorry he feels so sad.

10. A bird infected with the West Nile virus is bitten by a certain type of mosquito. The virus can then be transmitted to other birds and to humans by the mosquito. In this chain of infection, the mosquito is the:
    a. reservoir.
    b. vector.
    c. host.
    d. infectious agent.

11. The nurse writes the following expected outcome on the nursing care plan for a client who is diagnosed with a cerebral vascular accident: "The nurse will assist the client to the chair for meals every day." In applying the nursing process, this expected outcome:
    a. is written appropriately.
    b. is not measurable.
    c. should be client focused.
    d. should include how long the client may be in the chair.

12. The nurse is caring for a client who is incontinent of urine. Which nursing intervention is most effective in helping to maintain skin integrity?
    a. Change the incontinence pad q2h and prn.
    b. Limit liquid intake to 1000 mL per day.
    c. Insert an indwelling urinary catheter.
    d. Encourage daily intake of cranberry juice.

13. The nurse receives the following order for a client who is 1 day postop transurethral resection of the prostrate: "Irrigate the urinary catheter with NS 0.9% until free of clots." To appropriately implement this order, the nurse would:
    a. instill 100 mL of NS 0.9% every 2 hours into the urinary catheter.
    b. manually irrigate the catheter when clots are visible in the tubing.
    c. clarify the order to include the amount of NS to use.
    d. use clean technique to irrigate the catheter.

14. The nurse is caring for an elderly client just admitted with bronchopneumonia. Which client assessment finding is of greatest concern?
    a. Respirations 26
    b. Bilateral rhonchi
    c. Acute confusion
    d. Yellow-colored sputum

15. The nursing assistant informs the registered nurse that an elderly client, recovering from a cerebral vascular accident, had some difficulty swallowing during breakfast and choked on some food. In monitoring the client for the remainder of the shift, which assessment finding requires immediate follow-up?
    a. Pulse oximetry 98%
    b. 50% oral intake at noon
    c. Pulse 96 at noon; pulse 88 at 0800
    d. Temp 99.6° F at noon; temp 98.6° F at 0800

16. A client had a suprapubic catheter removed 2 days ago and is now being discharged. What is most important for the nurse to include in the discharge teaching?
    a. Urinary incontinence is normal for 1 to 2 weeks.
    b. Practice Kegel exercises five times per day.
    c. Empty the bladder every 2 to 3 hours for the first week.
    d. Limit fluid intake for the first week.

17. The nurse is delegating the care of a client who is 1 day postop to the nursing assistant. The nursing assistant asks whether the client's sequential stockings can be removed during the bath. Which response is most appropriate?
    a. "Do not remove the sequential stockings until tomorrow."
    b. "The sequential stockings can be removed while bathing the client."
    c. "Turn off the compression control device but do not remove the sequential stockings."
    d. "Remove the sequential stocking as you begin to wash each leg, but reapply them immediately."

18. The nurse receives an order for bladder training for a client who has an indwelling urinary catheter. The order reads: "Clamp catheter for 2 hours, then unclamp to empty bladder, then reclamp for 2 hours." After clamping the catheter for 1 hour, the client complains of bladder discomfort and indicates a 6/10 pain level. The nurse performs a bladder scan, which shows 150 mL of urine in the bladder. Which nursing action is most appropriate initially?
    a. Unclamp the catheter and allow the bladder to empty.
    b. Review the medication record for any pain medications.
    c. Reassess the amount of urine in the bladder in 15 minutes.
    d. Inform the client of the importance of maintaining the bladder training schedule.

19. The nurse is reading the nursing care plan of a client and notices that the expected outcome was for the client to eat 90% of the regular diet by today. The handoff report indicates that the client has been eating 50% of each meal for the last 24 hours. Which action by the nurse is most appropriate initially?
    a. Request the family bring in foods that the client likes.
    b. Assess the current needs of the client.
    c. Provide the client with between-meal snacks.
    d. Validate that the documentation in the chart is correct.

20. In the handoff report, the nurse learns that the assigned client has a Cheyne-Stokes breathing pattern. Which of the following would the nurse expect to see? (Select all that apply.)
    a. Periods of apnea
    b. Deep rapid breathing
    c. Shallow breathing
    d. Respiratory rate of 12 or less
    e. Full inspiration and expiration

21. The nurse is assigned to a client who receives furosemide 40 mg po BID direct IVP and digoxin 0.25 mg po qAM. To administer the morning dose of these drugs safely, the nurse should do which of the following? (Select all that apply.)
    a. Hold the digoxin if there are complaints of blurred vision.
    b. Monitor for signs of increased serum Na⁺ level.
    c. Hold the drugs if diuresis noted.
    d. Monitor for symptoms of decreased serum K⁺ level.
    e. Take the apical pulse for 30 seconds and multiply by 2.

22. A client is 4 days postop right total hip replacement with a cemented prosthesis. To prevent right hip dislocation, it is important to tell the client which of the following? (Select all that apply.)
    a. Bend at the waist to pick up items.
    b. Do not apply any weight on the right leg.
    c. Use an elevated toilet seat.
    d. Do not cross legs.
    e. Avoid lying on the right hip.

23. The nurse is caring for a client who is 3 days postop abdominal surgery. On changing the abdominal dressing, the nurse notes the surgical incision has eviscerated. The nurse is correct in doing which of the following? (Select all that apply.)
    a. Keep the client on bed rest.
    b. Apply a dry sterile dressing on the wound.
    c. Monitor vital signs q2h.
    d. Place a moist sterile dressing on the wound.
    e. Encourage fluid intake.

24. The nurse is assigned to care for a client diagnosed with diabetes mellitus type 1. The physician orders Lantus insulin 22 units qPM, fingerstick blood glucose testing AC and HS, and a correction bolus insulin scale (sliding scale) with Humulin R insulin. To appropriately implement the correction bolus insulin order, the nurse will plan to administer the Humulin R insulin (select all that apply)
    a. every time the fingerstick blood glucose is tested
    b. on the basis of the fingerstick blood glucose results
    c. 30 minutes after each meal and at the hour of sleep
    d. in combination with the Lantus insulin PM dose
    e. 5 units before each meal and at the hour of sleep

25. The nurse admits an adult client diagnosed with a bowel obstruction. The physician writes the following orders: (1) NPO, (2) insert a nasogastric tube to low wall suction. To implement the orders, the nurse would do which of the following? (Select all that apply.)
    a. Use a 10 F nasogastric tube
    b. Use a 14 F nasogastric tube
    c. Provide the client with water during insertion of the nasogastric tube
    d. Manually aspirate all gastric contents immediately after nasogastric tube insertion
    e. Ensure that the nasogastric tube is connected to the suction equipment before inserting the tube

2-1 STANDARDS OF PROFESSIONAL PERFORMANCE

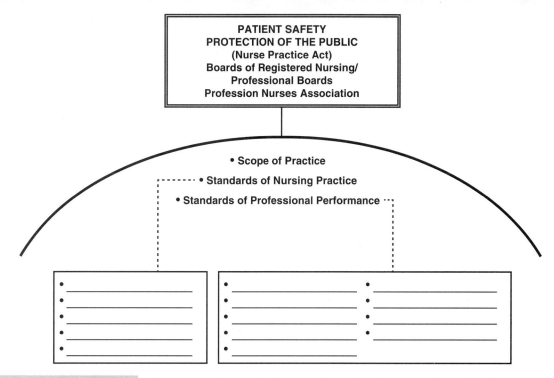

CLINICAL SITUATION   The RN on the medical-surgical unit has been a staff member for 15 years. She is clinically very competent and establishes good rapport with clients and their families. The RN has currently been assigned to work with nursing students. Several of the students have complained that it is difficult to work with this RN because she prefers to work independently and rarely answers the student's questions. The RN has commented to other staff that she only agreed to take students because the supervisor wants nursing students on the unit.

Pertinent Terminology	Definition
American Nurses Association (ANA)	
Canadian Nurses Association (CNA)	
Standards of Nursing Practice	
Standards of Professional Performance	

- Use the ANA Standards of Professional Performance to identify the behaviors that represent professional performance.
- Use the clinical situation to put an "X" in the middle column, which identifies the staff RN's professional performance behaviors that needs strengthening.

ANA Standards of Professional Performance		Write in behaviors that describe professional performance for each standard.
Quality of Practice		
Education		
Practice Evaluation		
Collegiality		
Collaboration		
Ethics		
Research		
Resource Utilization		
Leadership		

⚡ **Integrated Learning Activity:** With a partner, discuss the following statements related to "standards." __Underline__ the statements that are **TRUE.**

1. Standards, such as the Standards of Nursing Practice and Standards of Professional Practice, are considered legally binding regulations.

2. Standards of Nursing Practice can be used in a court of law in malpractice cases.

3. Standards of Nursing Practice identify the minimal expectations in the delivery of nursing care.

4. Professional nurses working in the outpatient setting are not held to the same standards of nursing practice as are professional nurses working in the acute care setting.

5. Additional standards of nursing care may be required in specialty areas such as medical-surgical units, pediatric units, and critical care units.

2-2 THE PATIENT UNDERGOING SURGERY (DEVELOPMENT OF SIGNS AND SYMPTOMS OF SHOCK)

Mr. H, age 60 years, was admitted with persistent abdominal pain. The baseline vital signs were T 99° F, P 98, R 20, BP 148/92. He states he has experienced nausea, vomiting, and a 10-pound weight loss within the last 2 months. He is diagnosed with gastric cancer and is scheduled for a subtotal gastrectomy in the morning. He has morphine sulfate 10 mg q3h direct IV injection prn, metoclopramide 10 mg direct IV injection q8h prn nausea, and Mylanta 30 mL po q2h prn abdominal pain. Mr. H is very anxious after speaking with his physician and refuses to sign the surgical consent. He tells the nurse that he is having abdominal pain and says his pain level is 10 out of 10 on the pain scale. He wants his pain shot "right now." The nurse notes that it is just about 3 hours since his last pain medication, and the Mylanta was given 2 hours ago.

Prioritize the following **nursing interventions** as you, the nurse, would do them to initially take care of Mr. H. Write a number in the box to identify the order of your interventions (#1 = first intervention, #2 = second intervention, etc.) and state a **rationale** for each intervention.

INTERVENTIONS	PRIORITY #	RATIONALE
• Administer IV pain med.	☐	_____
• Sit and talk with patient	☐	_____
• Give Mylanta 30 mL	☐	_____
• Offer to call a family member	☐	_____
• Notify physician	☐	_____

KEY POINTS TO CONSIDER _____

Mr. H does consent to have surgery and returns to the medical unit postoperatively. He has an IV of lactated Ringer's solution infusing at 125 mL/hr and you note the following:

1. P 90, R 20, BP 130/76
2. He is alert and oriented and his skin is warm and dry
3. NG tube draining brown-reddish drainage (300 mL in the last 4 hours)
4. Indwelling urinary catheter draining light yellow urine (700 mL in the last 4 hours)

Integrated Learning Activity: With a partner, **do the following: (1) on the basis of the current assessment, select** the **one nursing diagnosis** that is a priority at this time, **(2) provide a rationale** for your selection, and **(3) list three nursing interventions** that meet the needs of Mr. H:

All of the following nursing diagnoses may apply to Mr. H:

> Risk for infection, Acute pain, Anxiety, Ineffective airway clearance, Fatigue, Impaired physical mobility, Imbalanced nutrition: less than body requirements, Deficient knowledge, Risk for deficient fluid volume, Fear

Nursing Diagnosis	Rationale	Nursing Interventions

Several hours after surgery you note that Mr. H is very restless and you assess:
R 32, P 130, BP 108/70, NG drainage 200 mL bright red drainage, skin cool, c/o abdominal pain

Based on the situation, identify and write the **priority problem** in the box below. Then, starting with the small box labeled **#1, prioritize** the **nursing interventions** for this situation and identify your plan for follow-up care for Mr. H.

NURSING INTERVENTIONS

A. Monitor P, R, BP, and pulse oximetry

B. Document assessment/nursing care

C. Assess LOC and neuro status

D. Plan to start oxygen therapy

E. Stay with Mr. H

F. Notify physician

DECISION-MAKING DIAGRAM

New Action Plan

#1 #2 #3 #4 #5 #6

Priority Problem

NOTES _____

APPLYING CRITICAL THINKING SKILLS TO TEST QUESTIONS

INSTRUCTIONS: Circle the one best answer for each test question. Write your rationale for selecting the answer. To enhance your learning and test-taking skills, discuss your answer and rationale with a partner. The answer and the rationale can be found on the back of this page.

1. The nurse assesses the following on a client who had a colon resection 5 days ago: I & O × 4, skin warm, abdomen distended nontender, bowel sounds present. Abdominal sutures well approximated. States pain level 2 out of 10 on the pain scale. IV infusing at 75 mL/hr per pump. Fine crackles in the bilateral lower lung bases. In planning care, which nursing action is of priority?
   a. Take vital signs q4h
   b. Ambulate the client
   c. Assess lung sounds q4h
   d. Push oral fluids

   Rationale: _____
   _____
   _____
   _____
   _____

2. The nurse is caring for a client who has diabetes mellitus type 1 and is 2 days postop abdominal surgery. The client takes clopidrogrel (Plavix) 75 mg po daily and aspirin 81 mg po daily. In preparing the administration of these drugs, it is most important for the nurse to first:
   a. assess whether the client is having mild pain.
   b. check the serum prothrombin time levels.
   c. monitor the blood pressure.
   d. ensure that the client has eaten.

   Rationale: _____
   _____
   _____
   _____
   _____

3. The nurse administers atropine 0.4 mg IM as ordered preop for surgery. Thirty minutes after administration, the client complains of a very dry mouth and has flushed dry skin with an oral temperature of 99° F and a pulse rate of 104. The most appropriate nursing action is for the nurse to:
   a. document the client's complaints.
   b. notify the physician.
   c. take the client's temperature in 1 hour.
   d. recognize that these are normal side effects of the drug.

   Rationale: _____
   _____
   _____
   _____
   _____

ANSWER KEY FOR
APPLYING CRITICAL THINKING SKILLS TO TEST QUESTIONS

HELPFUL HINTS: Read all test questions carefully. Identify key words in the question that will guide you in answering the question. In these test questions the **key words** to consider are **"priority," "most important,"** and **"most appropriate."** Compare your rationale with the one in the test question.

1. The nurse assesses the following on a client who had a colon resection 5 days ago: I & O × 4, skin warm, abdomen distended nontender, bowel sounds present. Abdominal sutures well approximated. States pain level 2 out of 10 on the pain scale. IV infusing at 75 mL/hr per pump. Fine crackles in the bilateral lower lung bases. In planning care, which nursing action is of priority?
   a. Take vital signs q4h
   b. Ambulate the client
   c. Assess lung sounds q4h
   d. Push oral fluids

   Rationale: ___The answer is (b). Assessment data indicate the need to ambulate the client to ease abdominal distention and enhance respiration and movement of secretions. Options (a), (c), and (d) are important but do not help the client with the priority problems.___

2. The nurse is caring for a client who has diabetes mellitus type 1 and is 2 days postop abdominal surgery. The client takes clopidrogrel (Plavix) 75 mg po daily and aspirin 81 mg po daily. In preparing the administration of these drugs, it is most important for the nurse to first:
   a. assess whether the client is having mild pain.
   b. check the serum prothrombin time levels.
   c. monitor the blood pressure.
   d. ensure that the client has eaten.

   Rationale: ___The answer is (b). Clopidogrel and aspirin both have anticoagulation properties. Coagulation studies should be monitored throughout therapy. Options (a), (c), and (d) do not address the most important intervention related to this drug therapy.___

3. The nurse administers atropine 0.4 mg IM as ordered preop for surgery. Thirty minutes after administration, the client complains of a very dry mouth and has flushed dry skin with an oral temperature of 99° F and a pulse rate of 104. The most appropriate nursing action is for the nurse to:
   a. document the client's complaints.
   b. notify the physician.
   c. take the client's temperature in 1 hour.
   d. recognize that these are normal side effects of the drug.

   Rationale: ___The answer is (b). Atropine is a cholinergic blocking agent. The client is manifesting symptoms of adverse effects. Options (a) and (c) are not the most important. There is a narrow margin between the side effects and the adverse effects of the drug. The nurse should research the drug literature before selecting option (d).___

2-3 THE PATIENT WITH AN INTESTINAL OBSTRUCTION (DEVELOPMENT OF SIGNS AND SYMPTOMS OF DEHYDRATION)

Mrs. W, 56 years old, is hospitalized with the diagnosis of small bowel obstruction. She has an NG tube to low continuous suction draining dark brown drainage and an IV of D5/0.45 NS with 30 mEq potassium chloride (KCl) infusing at 100 mL/hr. Her skin is warm and dry and her mucous membranes are dry. Her abdomen is distended with hyperactive bowel sounds in the right upper and lower quadrants. The nursing assistant reports that Mrs. W just vomited 100 mL of dark brown secretions.

Prioritize the following **nursing interventions** as you would do them to initially take care of Mrs. W. Write a number in the box to identify the order of your interventions (#1 = first intervention, #2 = second intervention, etc.) and state a **rationale** for each intervention.

INTERVENTIONS	PRIORITY #	RATIONALE
• Provide thorough mouth care	☐	_____
• Assess abdomen, measure abdominal girth	☐	_____
• Assess NG tube and suction	☐	_____
• Take the vital signs	☐	_____
• Ensure Mrs. W is in semi-Fowler position	☐	_____

KEY POINTS TO CONSIDER _____

_____

TWO

After 48 hours Mrs. W's abdomen is less distended and the current assessment findings include:

1. Hemoglobin 9.2 g, hematocrit 29%, K^+ 3.1 mEq , Na^+ 145 mEq
2. T 98.8° F, P 92, irregular, R 20, BP 152/94
3. NG tube draining dark brown drainage (250 mL in the last 8 hours)
4. Pain on a 1-10 scale = 4
5. No stool or passing of flatus, urine output last 24 hr 600 mL

⚡ **Integrated Learning Activity:** With a partner, **do the following: (1) based on the current assessment, select** the **one nursing diagnosis** that is a priority at this time, **(2) provide a rationale** for your selection, and **(3) list three nursing interventions** that meet the needs of Mrs. W.

All of the following nursing diagnoses may apply to Mrs. W:

Risk for infection, Acute pain, Anxiety, Ineffective airway clearance, Imbalanced nutrition: less than body requirements, Deficient knowledge, Deficient fluid volume, Risk for impaired skin integrity, Fear, Disturbed sleep pattern

Nursing Diagnosis	Rationale	Nursing Interventions

The next day, Mrs. W's assessment included the following: NG output 500 mL and urine output 100 mL dark amber during the night shift. Faint bowel sounds, capillary refill >5 seconds. Weak, lethargic, and disoriented. Mucous membranes dry. Orthostatic BP 148/90 (lying), 124/84 (sitting).

On the basis of the situation, identify and write the **priority problem** in the box below. Then, starting with the small box labeled **#1, prioritize** the **nursing interventions** for this situation and identify your follow-up action plan for Mrs. W.

NURSING INTERVENTIONS   DECISION-MAKING DIAGRAM

A. Monitor IV fluid replacement

B. Inform physician

C. Orient Mrs. W

D. Provide oral care

E. Raise side rails

F. Take vital signs

New Action Plan

#1   #2   #3   #4   #5   #6

Priority Problem

NOTES _____

APPLYING CRITICAL THINKING SKILLS TO TEST QUESTIONS

INSTRUCTIONS: Circle the one best answer for each test question. Write your rationale for selecting the answer. To enhance your learning and test-taking skills, discuss your answer and rationale with a partner. The answer and the rationale can be found on the back of this page.

1. The nurse is taking care of a client who has an NG tube to continuous low suction. The nursing assistant reports that the client has vomited 100 mL of light yellow-greenish fluid. It is most important for the nurse to initially:
   a. check the medication record for an antiemetic.
   b. check NG tube placement.
   c. add the emesis to the total output for the shift.
   d. ask the client whether the desire to vomit has stopped.

   Rationale: _____
   _____
   _____
   _____
   _____

2. The nurse is caring for a client who was admitted with upper gastrointestinal bleeding. The client has an NG tube to continuous low suction and has an order for pantoprazole suspension 40 mg by NG tube daily. The nurse administers the medication at 0900. A priority follow-up nursing intervention is to:
   a. maintain the tube to low continuous suction.
   b. document medication administration.
   c. ensure NG tube placement.
   d. clamp the NG tube for 30 minutes.

   Rationale: _____
   _____
   _____
   _____
   _____

3. The client is receiving continuous full-strength formula tube feeding through an NG feeding tube at 75 mL/hr and there are 100 mL left in the feeding bag. The nurse is preparing to administer the 0900 routine medications through the feeding tube. Which technique is best for administering the 0900 medications?
   a. Crush the medications, dissolve in water, and put in the feeding bag.
   b. Crush the medications, dissolve in water, and give with a 50-mL syringe.
   c. Crush the medications, dissolve in water, and check tube placement.
   d. Crush the medications, dissolve in water, and check residual before giving.

   Rationale: _____
   _____
   _____
   _____
   _____

ANSWER KEY FOR
APPLYING CRITICAL THINKING SKILLS TO TEST QUESTIONS

HELPFUL HINTS: Read all test questions carefully. Identify key words in the question that will guide you in answering the question. In these test questions the **key words** to consider are **"most important," "priority,"** and **"best."** Compare your rationale with the one found for each question.

1. The nurse is taking care of a client who has an NG tube to continuous low suction. The nursing assistant reports that the client has vomited 100 mL of light yellow-greenish fluid. It is most important for the nurse to initially:
   a. check the medication record for an antiemetic.
   b. check NG tube placement.
   c. add the emesis to the total output for the shift.
   d. ask the client whether the desire to vomit has stopped.

   Rationale: The answer is (b). Vomiting should not be experienced with the use of an NG tube. Tube placement should be assessed. Option (a) is not the initial intervention and options (c) and (d) are not the most important interventions.

2. The nurse is caring for a client who was admitted with upper gastrointestinal bleeding. The client has an NG tube to continuous low suction and has an order for pantoprazole suspension 40 mg by NG tube daily. The nurse administers the medication at 0900. A priority follow-up nursing intervention is to:
   a. maintain the tube to low continuous suction.
   b. document medication administration.
   c. ensure NG tube placement.
   d. clamp the NG tube for 30 minutes.

   Rationale: The answer is (d). It is important to clamp the tube for 30 minutes to allow for drug absorption. Option (a) is an ongoing nursing action, option (b) should be done after drug administration, and option (c) should have been done before drug administration.

3. The client is receiving continuous full-strength formula tube feeding through an NG feeding tube at 75 mL/hr and there are 100 mL left in the feeding bag. The nurse is preparing to administer the 0900 routine medications through the feeding tube. Which technique is best for administering the 0900 medications?
   a. Crush the medications, dissolve in water, and put in the feeding bag.
   b. Crush the medications, dissolve in water, and give with a 50-mL syringe.
   c. Crush the medications, dissolve in water, and check tube placement.
   d. Crush the medications, dissolve in water, and check residual before giving.

   Rationale: The answer is (c). Tube placement should be checked before administration of medication or formula feeding. Options (a), (b), and (d) do not describe the best technique.

2-4 THE PATIENT WITH A COLOSTOMY
(DEVELOPMENT OF SIGNS AND SYMPTOMS OF STOMAL ISCHEMIA)

Mrs. P, 42 years old, had surgery today for colon cancer. She was transferred to her room 2 hours ago. In the evening handoff shift report you learn that she had a sigmoid colostomy and has a colostomy bag in place with the stoma edematous and red. The surgical dressing is clean and dry. The NG tube is to low continuous wall suction draining dark brown drainage. She has a right double lumen central line with total parenteral nutrition (TPN) infusing at 83 mL/hr, and an IV of D5/NS with a PCA (morphine sulfate) set to deliver 1 mg/6 min per patient demand, not to exceed 30 mg in 4 hours. Her latest VS: T98° F, P 86, R 18, BP 132/88, pain level 3 out of 10 on the pain scale. She is sleeping but easily arousable. Sequential stockings are on. There is an order for her to sit up at the side of the bed this evening. The morning lab work includes a CBC.

Prioritize the following **nursing interventions** as you, the nurse, would do them to initially take care of Mrs. P. Write a number in the box to identify the order of your interventions (#1 = first intervention, #2 = second intervention, etc.) and state a **rationale** for each intervention.

INTERVENTIONS	PRIORITY #	RATIONALE
• Assess surgical dressing and stoma	☐	_____
• Take the vital signs	☐	_____
• Assess pain level	☐	_____
• Check NG tube and drainage	☐	_____
• Check IV site, TPN, and PCA setting	☐	_____

KEY POINTS TO CONSIDER _____

The **first postop day** assessment was significant for the following signs and symptoms:
1. Bowel sounds absent
2. Mrs. P moans when she turns in bed
3. Weak, ineffective cough
4. Stoma swollen and reddened

⚡ **Integrated Learning Activity:** With a partner, **do the following: (1) select** the **one nursing diagnosis** that is a priority at this time, **(2) provide a rationale** for your selection, and **(3) list three nursing interventions** that assist you to meet the needs of the patient:

All of the following nursing diagnoses may apply to Mrs. P:

Risk for infection, Risk for impaired skin integrity, Acute pain, Anxiety, Ineffective airway clearance, Fatigue, Delayed surgical recovery, Imbalanced nutrition: less than body requirements, Disturbed body image, Risk for deficient fluid volume, Fear

Nursing Diagnosis	Rationale	Nursing Interventions

On the morning of the **third postop day,** the NG tube was removed per the physician's order, and Mrs. P was started on a clear liquid diet. In the afternoon the assessment findings included: stoma edematous and dusky, abdomen distended, pain level 8 out of 10 on the pain scale.

On the basis of the **third postop day** assessment, identify and write the **priority problem** in the box below. Then, starting with the small box labeled **#1,** **prioritize** the **nursing interventions** listed and **identify** your action plan for the follow-up care of Mrs. P.

NURSING INTERVENTIONS

A. Take the vital signs

B. Prepare to insert NG tube

C. Assess colostomy bag and bowel sounds

D. Notify physician stat

E. Place on NPO

F. Check IV patency

DECISION-MAKING DIAGRAM

New Action Plan

#1 #2 #3 #4 #5 #6

Priority Problem

NOTES _____

APPLYING CRITICAL THINKING SKILLS TO TEST QUESTIONS

INSTRUCTIONS: Circle the one best answer for each test question. Write your rationale for selecting the answer. To enhance your learning and test-taking skills, discuss your answer and rationale with a partner. The answer and the rationale can be found on the back of this page.

1. The handoff report of a client indicates that a double-barrel colostomy was performed 2 days ago. Which assessment finding is of most concern?
   a. Right-sided colostomy bag with small amount fecal drainage, left-sided colostomy bag with serosanguineous mucous drainage.
   b. Right-sided colostomy bag with serosanguineous mucous drainage. Stoma dark red. Left-sided colostomy bag with minimal drainage.
   c. Abdomen soft, tender to touch, stomas red and edematous.
   d. Bowel sounds hypoactive on right side; absent on left side.

   Rationale: _____
   _____
   _____
   _____
   _____

2. The nurse is assigned to a client who was had an ileostomy 3 days ago and is now started on a clear liquid diet. The client is receiving IV fluid set at 75 mL/hr. Which of the following interventions is most important for the nurse to ask the nursing assistant to perform?
   a. Take vital signs q4h
   b. Monitor intake and output q8h
   c. Give 500 mL of fluids for the shift
   d. Assist the client to turn in bed q4h

   Rationale: _____
   _____
   _____
   _____
   _____

3. The client is 72 years old and is admitted with a respiratory tract infection. The client is on erythromycin 400 mg q6h po. The client has a sigmoid colostomy. Which of the following assessment findings would be most indicative of a potential complication?
   a. Admission white blood cell count of 11,500
   b. Six liquid stools during the shift
   c. T 100.8° F during morning assessment
   d. Urinary output of 260 mL for the last 4 hours

   Rationale: _____
   _____
   _____
   _____
   _____

ANSWER KEY FOR
APPLYING CRITICAL THINKING SKILLS TO TEST QUESTIONS

HELPFUL HINTS: Read all test questions carefully. Identify key words in the question that will guide you in answering the question. In these test questions the **key words** to consider are **"most concern," "most important,"** and **"most indicative."** Compare your rationale with the one found for each question.

1. The handoff report of a client indicates that a double-barrel colostomy was performed 2 days ago. Which assessment finding is of most concern?
   a. Right-sided colostomy bag with small amount fecal drainage, left-sided colostomy bag with serosanguineous mucous drainage.
   b. Right-sided colostomy bag with serosanguineous mucous drainage. Stoma dark red. Left-sided colostomy bag with minimal drainage.
   c. Abdomen soft, tender to touch, stomas red and edematous.
   d. Bowel sounds hypoactive on right side; absent on left side.

   Rationale: The answer is (b). The dark red color of the stoma is an indication of possible impaired perfusion of the stoma. Options (a), (c), and (d) are normal assessment findings consistent with the situation.

2. The nurse is assigned to a client who was had an ileostomy 3 days ago and is now started on a clear liquid diet. The client is receiving IV fluid set at 75 mL/hr. Which of the following interventions is most important for the nurse to ask the nursing assistant to perform?
   a. Take vital signs q4h
   b. Monitor intake and output q8h
   c. Give 500 mL of fluids for the shift
   d. Assist the client to turn in bed q4h

   Rationale: The answer is (c). A new ileostomy will initially drain up to 2 L/day. Replacing fluid to prevent dehydration is important. Options (a), (b), and (d) are good interventions, but the client needs hydration because of the fluid loss.

3. The client is 72 years old and is admitted with a respiratory tract infection. The client is on erythromycin 400 mg q6h po. The client has a sigmoid colostomy. Which of the following assessment findings would be most indicative of a potential complication?
   a. Admission white blood cell count of 11,500
   b. Six liquid stools during the shift
   c. T 100.8° F during morning assessment
   d. Urinary output of 260 mL for the last 4 hours

   Rationale: The answer is (b). Erythromycin can cause diarrhea. With a sigmoid colostomy the client should have near-to-normal stools. Options (a) and (c) are symptoms associated with an infection, for which the client was admitted. Option (d) is within normal limits.

2-5 THE PATIENT WITH COLON CANCER (DEVELOPMENT OF SIGNS AND SYMPTOMS OF A VENOUS THROMBUS)

Mr. S, 65 years old, has colon cancer. He is admitted for a colon resection. His current medical history is significant for complaints of changes in bowel habits/constipation, passing of bloody stools, abdominal pain, and weight loss. His past medical condition includes a history of coronary artery disease and hypertension. In addition to antihypertensive medication, he takes aspirin 81 mg po daily. He indicates that he stopped this medication 3 days ago as recommended by his physician. In preparation for surgery, his current orders include NPO, insert an NG tube, and a saline lock. His 6:00 AM vital signs are T 98° F, P 78, R 20, BP 162/90, pain level 3 "abdominal cramping." He is to receive his preop medication at 12:00 noon today. The nurse receives the handoff report at 8:00 AM.

Prioritize the five **nursing interventions** as you, the nurse, would do them to initially take care of Mr. S. Write a number in the box to identify the order of your interventions (#1 = first intervention, #2 = second intervention, etc.) and state a **rationale** for each intervention.

INTERVENTIONS	PRIORITY #	RATIONALE
• Perform a body systems assessment	☐	_____ _____ _____
• Take the vital signs	☐	_____ _____ _____
• Insert saline lock	☐	_____ _____ _____
• Insert NG tube	☐	_____ _____ _____
• Check surgical consent	☐	_____ _____ _____

KEY POINTS TO CONSIDER _____

_____

_____

A colon resection is done on Mr. S. The **first postop day** assessment includes:
1. Lactated Ringer's infusing at 100 mL/hr and PCA with morphine sulfate
2. Elastic stockings on; intermittent compression device ordered for 24 hours
3. NG tube to low continuous wall suction draining brown-greenish fluid
4. Wants to stay in a low Fowler position
5. Short and shallow respirations

⚡ **Integrated Learning Activity:** With a partner, **do the following: (1)** based on the **first post-op day assessment, select the one nursing diagnosis** that is a priority at this time, **(2) provide a rationale** for your selection, and **(3) list three nursing interventions** that meet the needs of Mr. S.

All of the following nursing diagnoses may apply to Mr. S:

Risk for infection, Acute pain, Anxiety, Ineffective airway clearance, Imbalanced nutrition: less than body requirements, Deficient knowledge, Risk for deficient fluid volume, Risk for impaired skin integrity, Risk for ineffective peripheral tissue perfusion, Fear

Nursing Diagnosis	Rationale	Nursing Interventions

On the **fourth postoperative day,** you assess the following signs and symptoms on Mr. S:
• Complaints of tenderness in the right calf with a positive Homans' sign
• 2+ right ankle/calf edema; no edema noted on left ankle/calf
• Right calf is warmer to touch than the left calf

Based on the **fourth postoperative day** assessment, identify and write the **priority problem** in the box below. Then, starting with the small box labeled **#1,** prioritize the **nursing interventions** listed and **identify** your action plan for the follow-up care of Mr. S.

NURSING INTERVENTIONS   DECISION-MAKING DIAGRAM

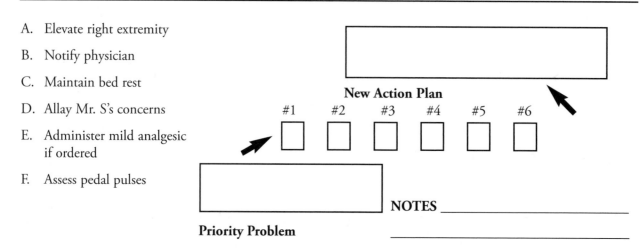

A. Elevate right extremity

B. Notify physician

C. Maintain bed rest

D. Allay Mr. S's concerns

E. Administer mild analgesic if ordered

F. Assess pedal pulses

New Action Plan

#1   #2   #3   #4   #5   #6

Priority Problem

NOTES _____

APPLYING CRITICAL THINKING SKILLS TO TEST QUESTIONS

INSTRUCTIONS: Circle the one best answer for each test question. Write your rationale for selecting the answer. To enhance your learning and test-taking skills, discuss your answer and rationale with a partner. The answer and the rationale can be found on the back of this page.

1. The nurse is caring for a client who had a ileostomy 5 days ago. The ileostomy is draining large amounts of green-brownish liquid stool. On discharge, the client asks the nurse whether the stool consistency will eventually become more solid. Which response by the nurse is best?
   a. "The stool will become solid as the ileostomy heals."
   b. "Eating certain foods can help make the stool more solid."
   c. "It takes about 1 year to see exactly what the stool consistency will be."
   d. "The stool will change to a mushy consistency after several months."

   Rationale: _____
   _____
   _____
   _____
   _____

2. The nurse is providing discharge instructions to a client who is going home after having an ileostomy for colon cancer. A priority discharge instruction is to instruct the client to:
   a. irrigate the ileostomy weekly.
   b. drink eight glasses of water daily.
   c. monitor the daily output from the ileostomy.
   d. use a mild laxative if there is no ileostomy drainage for 24 hours.

   Rationale: _____
   _____
   _____
   _____
   _____

3. The nurse is assisting a client to irrigate his colostomy. After instilling the water, the client has no output. What should the nurse do next?
   a. Encourage the client to ambulate
   b. Irrigate the colostomy again within 30 minutes
   c. Digitally stimulate the colostomy opening
   d. Notify the physician

   Rationale: _____
   _____
   _____
   _____
   _____

ANSWER KEY FOR
APPLYING CRITICAL THINKING SKILLS TO TEST QUESTIONS

HELPFUL HINTS: Read all test questions carefully. Identify key words in the question that will guide you in answering the question. In these test questions the **key words** to consider are **"best," "priority,"** and **"next."** Compare your rationale with the one in the test question.

1. The nurse is caring for a client who had a ileostomy 5 days ago. The ileostomy is draining large amounts of green-brownish liquid stool. On discharge, the client asks the nurse whether the stool consistency will eventually become more solid. Which response by the nurse is best?
   a. "The stool will become solid as the ileostomy heals."
   b. "Eating certain foods can help make the stool more solid."
   c. "It takes about 1 year to see exactly what the stool consistency will be."
   d. "The stool will change to a mushy consistency after several months."

   Rationale: The answer is (d). Fecal drainage from an ileostomy is mostly liquid and changes to a mushy consistency in 3 to 6 months. Options (a), (b), and (c) do not provide the client with the correct information.

2. The nurse is providing discharge instructions to a client who is going home after having an ileostomy for colon cancer. A priority discharge instruction is to instruct the client to:
   a. irrigate the ileostomy weekly.
   b. drink eight glasses of water daily.
   c. monitor the daily output from the ileostomy.
   d. use a mild laxative if there is no ileostomy drainage for 24 hours.

   Rationale: The answer is (b). Daily fecal drainage from a new ileostomy can range from 1000 to 2000 mL. The client is at risk for dehydration along with fluid and electrolyte imbalance. Options (a) and (d) are interventions that do not apply to the care of an ileostomy. Option (c) is good but does not help the client prevent a complication.

3. The nurse is assisting a client to irrigate his colostomy. After instilling the water, the client has no output. What should the nurse do next?
   a. Encourage the client to ambulate
   b. Irrigate the colostomy again within 30 minutes
   c. Digitally stimulate the colostomy opening
   d. Notify the physician

   Rationale: The answer is (a). Ambulation can stimulate peristalsis and the flow of fecal drainage. Option (b) would instill more fluid and may cause trauma and excessive loss of fluid and electrolytes. Option (c) is not appropriate and option (d) is not necessary because it may take some time for the drainage to begin.

2-6 THE PATIENT WITH TOTAL PARENTERAL NUTRITION (DEVELOPMENT OF SIGNS AND SYMPTOMS OF PULMONARY EMBOLUS)

You are assigned to care for Mrs. F. In the handoff report you learn that her diarrhea is decreasing and her current vital signs are T 98.8° F, P 76, R 18, BP 140/94, pulse ox 95%. She complained of pain in her right leg at a pain level of 3, no edema noted, pedal pulse is present.

VS q4h I & O (✓) Weigh qAM BRP with assist prn Admit date: 3/16 Name: F. J. M. Age: 55	Right central line inserted 3/16 Parenteral nutrition (PN) per IV pump @ 83 mL/hr Lipids 10% (M-W-F) infuse over 12 hours BG fingersticks q6h (6-12-6-12) Dx: Dehydration/Diarrhea Hx of Crohn—acute exacerbation, atrial fibrillation	Diet: NPO Routine med: Vit. K 10 mg subcut qMon Humulin Regular insulin 2 units if BG = 180 – 200 Call MD if BG more than 200

Prioritize the five **nursing interventions** as you would do them to take care of Mrs. F. Write a number in the box to identify the order of your interventions (#1 = first intervention, #2 = second intervention, etc.) and state a **rationale** for each intervention.

INTERVENTIONS	PRIORITY #	RATIONALE
• Perform a body systems physical assessment	☐	_____
• Assess right leg	☐	_____
• Assess central line for patency and central line dressing	☐	_____
• Get 0600 blood glucose results	☐	_____
• Assess right arm and neck for distention	☐	_____

KEY POINTS TO CONSIDER _____

Mrs. F was taken to x-ray 1 hour ago. On her return to the unit, the IV pump is beeping and you are informed that the machine has been beeping for a long time. You assess the following:

1. PN not infusing
2. Skin warm, diaphoretic, complains of nervousness and rapid heartbeat
3. VS: T 98° F, P 118, R 26, BP 136/90, pulse ox 96%

Integrated Learning Activity: With a partner, **do the following: (1) select** the **one nursing diagnosis** that is a priority at this time, **(2) provide a rationale** for your selection, and **(3) list the nursing interventions** that assist you to meet the needs of the patient:

All of the following nursing diagnoses may apply to Mrs. F:

Anxiety, Risk for infection, Risk for activity intolerance, Imbalanced fluid volume, Impaired tissue integrity, Ineffective peripheral tissue perfusion, Imbalanced nutrition: less than body requirements, Risk for injury: hypoglycemia, Deficient knowledge

Nursing Diagnosis	Rationale	Nursing Interventions

Three hours later, Mrs. F's family comes to the nursing station to say that Mrs. F is having difficulty breathing. You go into Mrs. F's room and assess the following: complaints of chest pain, R 36, P 134, BP 108/88, pulse ox 90%, coughing, dyspnea, anxiousness.

On the basis of the situation **3 hours later**, identify and write the **priority problem** in the box below. Then, starting with the small box labeled **#1**, **prioritize** the **nursing interventions** for this situation and **identify** your follow-up action plan for Mrs. F.

NURSING INTERVENTIONS

A. Stay with Mrs. F
B. Raise head of bed
C. Take P, R, BP, assess pain level
D. Monitor oxygen saturation level
E. Notify MD
F. Administer oxygen

DECISION-MAKING DIAGRAM

New Action Plan

#1 #2 #3 #4 #5 #6

Priority Problem

NOTES _____

_____

TWO

2-7 THE PATIENT WITH CIRRHOSIS OF THE LIVER (DEVELOPMENT OF SIGNS AND SYMPTOMS INDICATIVE OF BLEEDING TENDENCY)

Mr. U, 46 years old, was admitted with the diagnosis of Laënnec's cirrhosis. In the handoff evening report you learn that he is jaundiced, has ascites, and has increasing shortness of breath. His VS at 12:00 noon were T 99° F, P 94, R 34, BP 140/90, pulse ox 96%, pain level 0. The vital signs are consistent with previous recordings. The handoff report is completed at 4:30 PM. The nursing care Kardex (rand) includes the following orders:

| VS q4h   I & O (✓)
Neuro cks q4h

CBC, serum ammonia }
AST, ALT, PT } today

Procedure: Abd paracentesis at 5:00 PM today | Saline lock (✓)

Bed rest with BRP

Weigh daily
Measure abd girth daily | Diet: ↑ CHO, 30 g prot., 2 g Na⁺

Routine med:
Amphogel 30 mL po qid
Furosemide 40 mg IVP qAM
Aldactone 50 mg po bid |

Prioritize the five **nursing interventions** as you would do them to take care of Mr. U. Write a number in the box to identify the order of your interventions (#1 = first intervention, #2 = second intervention, etc.) and state a **rationale** for each intervention.

INTERVENTIONS	PRIORITY #	RATIONALE
• Ensure that consent form is signed	☐	_____
• Take the vital signs	☐	_____
• Perform a body systems physical assessment	☐	_____
• Ensure that abdominal paracentesis equipment is on the unit	☐	_____
• Have Mr. U void	☐	_____

KEY POINTS TO CONSIDER _____

The physician performs the abdominal paracentesis on Mr. U and removes 2.5 L of fluid. VS during the procedure were P 90, R 32, BP 136/86. Post procedure you assess:

1. VS: P 94, R 24, BP 136/86, pain level 1
2. Dressing at the abdominal puncture site is clean
3. Mr. U is lying in a semi-Fowler position
4. He is alert and oriented, although slow to respond

Integrated Learning Activity: With a partner, **do the following: (1) select** the **one nursing diagnosis** that is a priority at this time, **(2) provide a rationale** for your selection, and **(3) list the nursing interventions** that assist you to meet the needs of the patient.

All of the following nursing diagnoses may apply to Mr. U:

> Risk for falls, Risk for infection, Impaired skin integrity, Impaired physical mobility, Acute pain, Imbalanced nutrition: less than body requirements, Risk for activity intolerance, Impaired tissue integrity, Excess fluid volume, Risk for deficient fluid volume, Ineffective breathing pattern, Disturbed body image, Disturbed sleep pattern, Fatigue, Impaired comfort

Nursing Diagnosis	Rationale	Nursing Interventions

The **laboratory results** for today are:

PT 40 sec	Serum ammonia 70 mcg/dL	Hgb 10.6 g/dL	Hct 30%
WBC 3500/mm^3	Platelets 100,000/mm^3	AST 100 U/L	ALT 500 U/L

Based on the **laboratory results**, identify and write the **priority problem** in the box below. Then, starting with the small box labeled **#1, prioritize** the **nursing interventions** for this situation and **identify** your follow-up action plan for Mr. U.

NURSING INTERVENTIONS

A. Monitor the VS

B. Assess for petechiae

C. Check stool for occult blood

D. Monitor urine color

E. Check neuro status

F. Notify MD

DECISION-MAKING DIAGRAM

New Action Plan

#1 #2 #3 #4 #5 #6

Priority Problem

NOTES _____

TWO

APPLYING CRITICAL THINKING SKILLS TO TEST QUESTIONS

INSTRUCTIONS: Circle the one best answer for each test question. Write your rationale for selecting the answer. To enhance your learning and test-taking skills, discuss your answer and rationale with a partner. The answer and the rationale can be found on the back of this page.

1. The physicians order phytonadione (vitamin K) 10 mg IM for an adult client with liver cirrhosis and ascites. Available is a vial of phytonadione 10 mg/mL. The nurse is planning to administer this dose in the deltoid. Which of the following is most appropriate for the administration of the ordered amount to the client?
   a. 1-mL syringe with 25-gauge ⅝-inch needle
   b. 1-mL syringe with 23-gauge ½-inch needle
   c. 3-mL syringe with 23-gauge 1-inch needle
   d. 3-mL syringe with 22-gauge 1½-inch needle

   Rationale: _____
   _____
   _____
   _____
   _____

2. The nurse admits a client with cirrhosis of the liver and severe ascites. The client is oriented, jaundiced, and complains of itching. Respirations are 28, short and shallow. Urine is dark amber. Which action is most important for the nurse to consider?
   a. Sit client in high Fowler position.
   b. Encourage client to drink more fluids.
   c. Limit client activity.
   d. Assess skin integrity daily.

   Rationale: _____
   _____
   _____
   _____
   _____

3. The client is admitted with cirrhosis of the liver and ascites. The physician orders the administration of an IV infusion of albumin. Which of the following is the expected outcome after the administration of the albumin?
   a. Decreased complaints of pruritis
   b. Decreased serum ammonia levels
   c. Increased secretion of sodium
   d. Increased urinary output

   Rationale: _____
   _____
   _____
   _____
   _____

ANSWER KEY FOR
APPLYING CRITICAL THINKING SKILLS TO TEST QUESTIONS

HELPFUL HINTS: Read all test questions carefully. Identify key words in the question that will guide you in answering the question. In these test questions the **key words** to consider are **"most appropriate," "most important,"** and **"expected outcome."** Compare your rationale with the one in the test question.

1. The physicians order phytonadione (vitamin K) 10 mg IM for an adult client with liver cirrhosis and ascites. Available is a vial of phytonadione 10 mg/mL. The nurse is planning to administer this dose in the deltoid. Which of the following is most appropriate for the administration of the ordered amount to the client?
   a. 1-mL syringe with 25-gauge ⅝-inch needle
   b. 1-mL syringe with 23-gauge ½-inch needle
   c. 3-mL syringe with 23-gauge 1-inch needle
   d. 3-mL syringe with 22-gauge 1½-inch needle

   Rationale: The answer is (c). It is most appropriate to use a smaller IM needle gauge because clients with liver cirrhosis are at a high risk for bleeding. The deltoid is a smaller muscle than the gluteus, so a 1-inch needle is the best choice. Options (a), (b), and (d) are not the best choice for this client.

2. The nurse admits a client with cirrhosis of the liver and severe ascites. The client is oriented, jaundiced, and complains of itching. Respirations are 28, short and shallow. Urine is dark amber. Which action is most important for the nurse to consider?
   a. Sit client in high Fowler position.
   b. Encourage client to drink more fluids.
   c. Limit client activity.
   d. Assess skin integrity daily.

   Rationale: The answer is (c). Activity increases the metabolic needs of the body, thereby increasing the workload of the liver. Option (a) is not the most appropriate position for a client with severe ascites because it compromises respiration. Options (b) and (d) are not the most important interventions.

3. The client is admitted with cirrhosis of the liver and ascites. The physician orders the administration of an IV infusion of albumin. Which of the following is the expected outcome after the administration of the albumin?
   a. Decreased complaints of pruritis
   b. Decreased serum ammonia levels
   c. Increased secretion of sodium
   d. Increased urinary output

   Rationale: The answer is (d). Albumin increases plasma colloid osmotic pressure, thereby increasing diuresis. Options (a), (b), and (c) are not expected outcomes for this ordered intervention.

2-8 THE PATIENT WITH HEPATIC ENCEPHALOPATHY (DEVELOPMENT OF SIGNS AND SYMPTOMS INDICATIVE OF IMPENDING COMA)

TWO

Mr. U, 47 years old, is admitted with the diagnosis of hepatic encephalopathy related to his advanced cirrhosis of the liver. The 11-7 shift handoff report indicates that he was awake most of the night, very restless, and confused to time and place. VS at 0400 were T 97° F Ax, P 88, R 22, BP 120/88, pulse ox 92%. The nurse states that she was unable to assess pain level but made every effort to keep him comfortable. The nursing care Kardex has the following orders:

VS q4 I & O (✓)	D_5W @ 100 mL/hr	Diet: ↑ CHO, 50 g Prot., 4 g Na^+
Neuro cks q4h	#20 g RFA – inserted today	Routine med:
Serum ammonia, K^+ today	Bed rest with BRP	Neomycin 1 g po q6h
Code status: No code	Weigh daily	Lactulose 30 mL bid

As you enter his room you notice that Mr. U is sleeping.

Prioritize the five **nursing interventions** as you would do them to take care of Mr. U. Write a number in the box to identify the order of your interventions (#1 = first intervention, #2 = second intervention, etc.) and state a **rationale** for each intervention.

INTERVENTIONS	PRIORITY #	RATIONALE
• Take VS	☐	_____
• Assess level of consciousness and orientation	☐	_____
• Check current serum ammonia and K^+ levels	☐	_____
• Perform a body systems physical assessment	☐	_____
• Assist Mr. U with his activities of daily living and provide comfort care	☐	_____

KEY POINTS TO CONSIDER _____

_____

Mr. U has refused his morning dose of lactulose and you further assess:
1. He refused the lactulose the previous day
2. No bowel movement for 2 days
3. Irritable, speech slurred
4. Responds slowly to verbal communication

Integrated Learning Activity: With a partner, **do the following: (1) select** the **one nursing diagnosis** that is a priority at this time, **(2) provide a rationale** for your selection, and **(3) list the nursing interventions** that assist you to meet the needs of the patient.

All of the following nursing diagnoses may apply to Mr. U:

> Risk for falls, Risk for infection, Impaired skin integrity, Bathing self-care deficit, Impaired physical mobility, Constipation, Imbalanced nutrition: less than body requirements, Activity intolerance, Impaired tissue integrity, Excess fluid volume, Ineffective breathing pattern, Fatigue, Disturbed sleep pattern, Impaired comfort

Nursing Diagnosis	Rationale	Nursing Interventions

You return from lunch at 1 PM and are informed of the following: Mr. U is becoming increasingly confused and lethargic. He did not eat lunch.

Based on the 1 PM information, identify and write the **priority problem** in the box below. Then, starting with the small box labeled **#1, prioritize** the **nursing interventions** for this situation and **identify** your follow-up action plan for Mr. U.

NURSING INTERVENTIONS

A. Inform physician

B. Document assessment findings

C. Take VS, pulse ox

D. Monitor neurologic status

E. Stay with patient

F. Raise the bedrails

DECISION-MAKING DIAGRAM

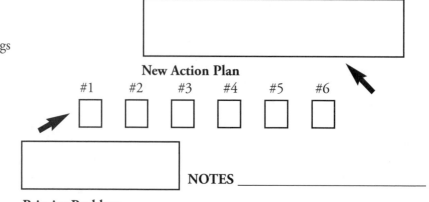

New Action Plan

#1   #2   #3   #4   #5   #6

Priority Problem

NOTES _____

APPLYING CRITICAL THINKING SKILLS TO TEST QUESTIONS

INSTRUCTIONS: Circle the one best answer for each test question. Write your rationale for selecting the answer. To enhance your learning and test-taking skills, discuss your answer and rationale with a partner. The answer and the rationale can be found on the back of this page.

1. The client is diagnosed with hepatic encephalopathy and is receiving lactulose 30 mL po bid. To effectively monitor the therapeutic effects of the drug therapy, the nurse would primarily assess for a(n):
   a. decrease in abdominal girth.
   b. increase in bowel movements.
   c. increase in serum albumin levels.
   d. decrease in serum ammonia levels.

   Rationale: _____

   _____

   _____

   _____

   _____

2. The nurse administers spironolactone 100 mg po to a client with portal hypertension. Which of the following is most important for the nurse to monitor during the administration of this drug?
   a. Serum potassium levels
   b. Intake and output
   c. Specific gravity of urine
   d. Abdominal girth

   Rationale: _____

   _____

   _____

   _____

   _____

3. The nurse is caring for a client admitted with portal hypertension and ascites. Which assessment finding is most indicative of a serious complication?
   a. Caput medusae noted on abdomen
   b. Complaints of fatigue and weakness
   c. Hematemesis after breakfast
   d. 2-pound weight loss from previous day

   Rationale: _____

   _____

   _____

   _____

   _____

ANSWER KEY FOR
APPLYING CRITICAL THINKING SKILLS TO TEST QUESTIONS

HELPFUL HINTS: Read all test questions carefully. Identify key words in the question that will guide you in answering the question. In these test questions the **key words** to consider are **"primarily," "most important,"** and **"most indicative."** Compare your rationale with the one in the test question.

1. The client is diagnosed with hepatic encephalopathy and is receiving lactulose 30 mL po bid. To effectively monitor the therapeutic effects of the drug therapy, the nurse would primarily assess for a(n):
   a. decrease in abdominal girth.
   b. increase in bowel movements.
   c. increase in serum albumin levels.
   d. decrease in serum ammonia levels.

   Rationale: _The answer is (d). The expected therapeutic effect for this client is to decrease serum ammonia levels by trapping ammonium ions in the intestine and excreting them in the stool. Options (a) and (c) do not provide the nurse with the therapeutic drug effects, and option (b) is not as specific a measure of effectiveness as the serum ammonia level._

2. The nurse administers spironolactone 100 mg po to a client with portal hypertension. Which of the following is most important for the nurse to monitor during the administration of this drug?
   a. Serum potassium levels
   b. Intake and output
   c. Specific gravity of urine
   d. Abdominal girth

   Rationale: _The answer is (a). Serum potassium levels should be monitored when a client is on spironolactone, a potassium-sparing diuretic. Options (b), (c), and (d) are not the most important interventions._

3. The nurse is caring for a client admitted with portal hypertension and ascites. Which assessment finding is most indicative of a serious complication?
   a. Caput medusae noted on abdomen
   b. Complaints of fatigue and weakness
   c. Hematemesis after breakfast
   d. 2-pound weight loss from previous day

   Rationale: _The answer is (c). Clients with portal hypertension may also have esophageal varices. The client should be monitored for further signs of bleeding. Option (a) is an expected finding consistent with ascites. Option (b) needs further assessment, and option (d) is not most indicative of a serious complication._

2-9 THE PATIENT WITH DIABETES MELLITUS (DEVELOPMENT OF A HYPOGLYCEMIC EPISODE)

The nurse is assigned to a 56-year-old Hispanic female, Mrs. G, admitted with the diagnosis of end-stage renal disease (ESRD). She has a 30-year history of type 1 diabetes mellitus and is scheduled to have hemodialysis this AM.

The handoff report included the following: VS: T 36° C, P 80, R 18, BP 154/92 pulse ox 94%, pain level 0. Mrs. G has a 2-cm dry, ulcerated circular area on the lateral outer aspect of her right great toe and an arteriovenous (AV) fistula in the right forearm. There is an order for Humulin N insulin 25 units subcut qAM and Humulin N 15 units in the evening. The blood glucose fingersticks are ordered ac and at 9:00 PM. It is 0730 when the handoff report is completed and breakfast arrives on the unit at 0800.

Prioritize the five **nursing interventions** as you would do them to initially take care of Mrs. G. Write a number in the box to identify the order of your interventions (#1 = first intervention, #2 = second intervention, etc.) and state a **rationale** for each intervention.

INTERVENTIONS	PRIORITY #	RATIONALE
• Check for the fingerstick blood glucose	☐	_____
• Assess AV fistula	☐	_____
• Administer Humulin N 25 units subcut	☐	_____
• Give patient the breakfast	☐	_____
• Perform a body systems physical assessment	☐	_____

KEY POINTS TO CONSIDER _____

Mrs. G is still waiting for her dialysis treatment. At 1000 the physician leaves the following orders:

Correction bolus insulin scale (sliding scale)   251-275 give 3 units Humalog insulin.
for fingerstick blood glucose: 211-250 give 2 units Humalog insulin.
150-210 give 1 unit Humalog insulin.
Less than 150 no insulin.

You do a BG fingerstick at 1145. The BG results are 215. You will give ___*2 units*___ Humalog insulin 15 minutes before lunch.

⚡ **Integrated Learning Activity:** With a partner, **do the following: (1) select** the **one nursing diagnosis** that is a priority at this time, **(2) provide a rationale** for your selection, and **(3) list the nursing interventions** that assist you to meet the needs of the patient.

All of the following nursing diagnoses may apply to Mrs. G:

Risk for infection, Risk for impaired skin integrity, Impaired physical mobility, Ineffective sexuality patterns, Fatigue, Excess fluid volume, Deficient fluid volume, Imbalanced nutrition: less than body requirements

Nursing Diagnosis	Rationale	Nursing Interventions
Excess fluid volume	*Renal disease*	*—*

As you take her 1300 VS, you note the following signs and symptoms: irritability, skin warm, moist, VS: T 36.8° C, P 100, R 18, BP 150/84. She complains of dizziness and "feeling funny." You suspect a hypo-glycemic reaction.

On the basis of the situation above, identify and write the **priority problem** in the box below. Then, starting with the small box labeled **#1, prioritize** the **nursing interventions** for this situation and **identify** your plan for follow-up care for Mrs. G.

NURSING INTERVENTIONS   **DECISION-MAKING DIAGRAM**

A. Document findings/nursing care

B. Do a fingerstick blood glucose stat

C. Check fingerstick blood glucose
in 15 minutes

New Action Plan

#1 #2 #3 #4 #5 #6
□   □   □   □   □   □

D. Prepare to give 4 ounces of
apple juice

E. Alert the RN stat

F. Raise the side rails

NOTES _____

Priority Problem

_____

APPLYING CRITICAL THINKING SKILLS TO TEST QUESTIONS

INSTRUCTIONS: Circle the one best answer for each test question. Write your rationale for selecting the answer. To enhance your learning and test-taking skills, discuss your answer and rationale with a partner. The answer and the rationale can be found on the back of this page.

1. The nurse is providing discharge instructions to a newly diagnosed client with type 1 diabetes mellitus who will take 5 units Humulin R insulin and 10 units Humulin N insulin qAM. The client informs the nurse that he runs 2 miles every morning. In teaching the client about insulin absorption and exercise, it is important for the nurse to teach the client to:
   a. inject the morning dose of insulin into the abdomen.
   b. hold the morning dose of Humulin R insulin until after the exercise.
   c. hold the morning dose of Humulin N insulin until after the exercise.
   d. inject the morning dose of insulin into the lower extremity.

   Rationale: _____
   _____
   _____
   _____
   _____

2. The nurse notes the following medications on a client's medication record: Humulin N insulin 13 units subcut qAM at 0730 and Humalog (lispro) 5 units subcut at the start of breakfast. The breakfast arrives at 0830 on the unit. In assessing the medication record, which action by the nurse is most appropriate?
   a. Question the Humalog (lispro) insulin order.
   b. Question the Humulin N insulin order.
   c. Give both insulins at 0730 in one syringe.
   d. Give the insulins as ordered.

   Rationale: _____
   _____
   _____
   _____
   _____

3. The nurse is preparing to draw up Lantus 12 units using a low-dose insulin syringe. Which technique indicates the most appropriate procedure before giving the insulin? The nurse takes the medication record and the insulin syringe with the 12 units of insulin and:
   a. checks the drawn-up dose with another nurse.
   b. with the syringe in the vial, checks the drawn-up dose with another nurse.
   c. takes the vial of insulin to check the drawn-up dose with another nurse.
   d. double-checks by charting the dose of insulin before injecting the insulin.

   Rationale: _____
   _____
   _____
   _____
   _____

ANSWER KEY FOR
APPLYING CRITICAL THINKING SKILLS TO TEST QUESTIONS

HELPFUL HINTS: Read all test questions carefully. Identify key words in the question that will guide you in answering the question. In these test questions the **key words** to consider are **"absorption and exercise"** and **"most appropriate."** Compare your rationale with the one in the test question.

1. The nurse is providing discharge instructions to a newly diagnosed client with type 1 diabetes mellitus who will take 5 units Humulin R insulin and 10 units Humulin N insulin qAM. The client informs the nurse that he runs 2 miles every morning. In teaching the client about insulin absorption and exercise, it is important for the nurse to teach the client to:
   a. inject the morning dose of insulin into the abdomen.
   b. hold the morning dose of Humulin R insulin until after the exercise.
   c. hold the morning dose of Humulin N insulin until after the exercise.
   d. inject the morning dose of insulin into the lower extremity.

   Rationale: _The answer is (a). The abdomen is a better injection site because the absorption rate of insulin is faster when injected into an extremity that is exercised. Options (b), (c), and (d) do not correlate the effects of diabetes, insulin therapy, and exercise._

2. The nurse notes the following medications on a client's medication record: Humulin N insulin 13 units subcut qAM at 0730 and Humalog (lispro) 5 units subcut at the start of breakfast. The breakfast arrives at 0830 on the unit. In assessing the medication record, which action by the nurse is most appropriate?
   a. Question the Humalog (lispro) insulin order.
   b. Question the Humulin N insulin order.
   c. Give both insulins at 0730 in one syringe.
   d. Give the insulins as ordered.

   Rationale: _The answer is (d). It is most appropriate to consider that Humalog (lispro) is a rapid-acting insulin with an onset of 10 to 15 minutes and should be administered at the start of the meal. Options (a), (b), and (c) do not address the onset of action of the rapid-acting insulin._

3. The nurse is preparing to draw up Lantus 12 units using a low-dose insulin syringe. Which technique indicates the most appropriate procedure before giving the insulin? The nurse takes the medication record and the insulin syringe with the 12 units of insulin and:
   a. checks the drawn-up dose with another nurse.
   b. with the syringe in the vial, checks the drawn-up dose with another nurse.
   c. takes the vial of insulin to check the drawn-up dose with another nurse.
   d. double-checks by charting the dose of insulin before injecting the insulin.

   Rationale: _The answer is (b). To prevent a medication error, it is recommended that the syringe remain in the insulin vial when checking the type and dose of insulin with another nurse. Options (a), (c), and (d) are not the most appropriate and recommended procedure._

2-10 THE PATIENT UNDERGOING HEMODIALYSIS (DEVELOPMENT OF SIGNS AND SYMPTOMS OF DISEQUILIBRIUM SYNDROME)

TWO

Ms. A, 52 years old, has ESRD and has just been started on dialysis. She has an AV fistula in the right forearm and is scheduled for dialysis at 0800 today. The handoff report is brief with only significant findings given: AV fistula has a strong thrill and bruit. Ms. A's BP is 160/102. Patient has not been weighed this morning. The report is completed at 0730 and you note the following orders from the nursing care Kardex:

VS q8h I & O (✓) Hemodialysis today Weigh daily Hgb & Hct (✓) Serum Ferritin (✓) Serum iron saturation (✓) Electrolytes (Na^+, K^+, CL^-, CO_2)	IV: Saline lock—left hand Routine medications: Enalapril 10 mg po qAM 0800 Folic acid 1 mg po qAM 0800 $FeSO_4$ 325 po tid c̄ meals Epoetin alfa 30,000 units subcut M-W-F	Diet: 70 g protein, 2 g Na^+, 2 g K^+ Fluid restriction 1000 mL/day

Prioritize the five **nursing interventions** as you would do them to take care of Ms. A. Write a number in the box to identify the order of your interventions (#1 = first intervention, #2 = second intervention, etc.) and state a **rationale** for each intervention.

INTERVENTIONS	PRIORITY #	RATIONALE
• Take the VS (BP on the left arm)	☐	_____
• Perform body systems physical assessment	☐	_____
• Weigh patient	☐	_____
• Assess AV fistula for thrill and bruit	☐	_____
• Hold folic acid and enalapril	☐	_____

KEY POINTS TO CONSIDER _____

Ordered laboratory studies were drawn before dialysis. The results of the morning laboratory tests are:
1. Hemoglobin 9.5 g/dL, hematocrit 28%
2. Ferritin 60 ng/mL
3. Serum iron saturation 18%
4. K+ 5.0 mEq

Integrated Learning Activity: With a partner, **do the following: (1) select** the **one nursing diagnosis** that is a priority at this time, **(2) provide a rationale** for your selection, and **(3) list the nursing interventions** that assist you to meet the needs of the patient.

All of the following nursing diagnoses may apply to Ms. A:

Risk for injury, Deficient knowledge, Fear, Anxiety, Risk for infection, Impaired tissue integrity, Constipation, Excess fluid volume, Deficient fluid volume, Disturbed body image, Impaired physical mobility, Ineffective peripheral tissue perfusion, Imbalanced nutrition: less than body requirements, Fatigue

Nursing Diagnosis	Rationale	Nursing Interventions

After the dialysis treatment, Ms. A is restless and you assess: Complains of headache, pruritus, nausea, change in level of consciousness, twitching, confusion

On the basis of data **after the dialysis treatment,** identify and write the **priority problem** in the box below. Then, starting with the small box labeled **#1, prioritize** the **nursing interventions** for this situation and **identify** your follow-up action plan for Ms. A.

NURSING INTERVENTIONS

A. Take the VS
B. Notify physician
C. Maintain calm, quiet environment
D. Stay with patient
E. Monitor neurologic status
F. Document assessment findings

DECISION-MAKING DIAGRAM

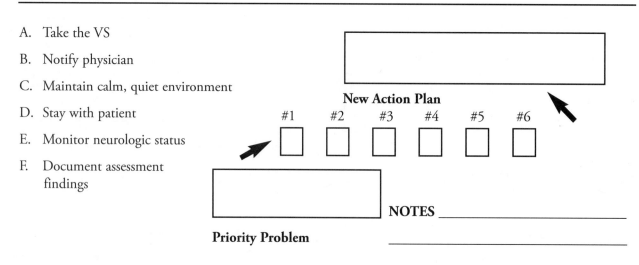

New Action Plan

#1 #2 #3 #4 #5 #6

Priority Problem

NOTES _____

_____

TWO

APPLYING CRITICAL THINKING SKILLS TO TEST QUESTIONS

INSTRUCTIONS: Circle the one best answer for each test question. Write your rationale for selecting the answer. To enhance your learning and test-taking skills, discuss your answer and rationale with a partner. The answer and the rationale can be found on the back of this page.

1. The client with ESRD related to type 1 diabetes mellitus has completed hemodialysis 1 hour ago. Which nursing intervention is of priority in assisting the alert adult client to transfer from the bed to the chair after dialysis?
   a. Check the blood glucose level.
   b. Monitor for dizziness on standing.
   c. Wrap the AV fistula with gauze.
   d. Do not move the arm with the AV fistula.

   Rationale: _____
   _____
   _____
   _____
   _____

2. The nurse administers epoetin alfa 10,000 units subcut twice weekly to the client with ESRD. The most effective method of evaluating the therapeutic effect of epoetin alfa is for the nurse to assess for:
   a. a decrease in skin pallor.
   b. an increase in client activity.
   c. an increase in the hematocrit level.
   d. a decrease in complaints of weakness and fatigue.

   Rationale: _____
   _____
   _____
   _____
   _____

3. The nurse is caring for a client scheduled for hemodialysis this morning. In preparing the client for the dialysis treatment, it is most important for the nurse to:
   a. allow the client to rest until after the dialysis treatment.
   b. ensure that all morning care is completed before dialysis.
   c. make the client NPO until after the dialysis treatment.
   d. withhold the morning dose of any antihypertensive drugs.

   Rationale: _____
   _____
   _____
   _____
   _____

ANSWER KEY FOR
APPLYING CRITICAL THINKING SKILLS TO TEST QUESTIONS

HELPFUL HINTS: Read all test questions carefully. Identify key words in the question that will guide you in answering the question. In these test questions the **key words** to consider are **"priority," "most effective,"** and **"most important."** Compare your rationale with the one in the test question.

1. The client with ESRD related to type 1 diabetes mellitus has completed hemodialysis 1 hour ago. Which nursing intervention is of priority in assisting the alert adult client to transfer from the bed to the chair after dialysis?
   a. Check the blood glucose level.
   b. Monitor for dizziness on standing.
   c. Wrap the AV fistula with gauze.
   d. Do not move the arm with the AV fistula.

   Rationale: ___The answer is (b). Hypotension is a postdialysis complication related to rapid removal of fluid. The nurse should monitor for orthostatic changes. Options (a) and (c) are important but not of priority after dialysis. Option (d) is an intervention that can apply to a new fistula.___

2. The nurse administers epoetin alfa 10,000 units subcut twice weekly to the client with ESRD. The most effective method of evaluating the therapeutic effect of epoetin alfa is for the nurse to assess for:
   a. a decrease in skin pallor.
   b. an increase in client activity.
   c. an increase in the hematocrit level.
   d. a decrease in complaints of weakness and fatigue.

   Rationale: ___The answer is (c). Epoetin alfa stimulates the production of red blood cells. The hematocrit is an indirect measurement of the total number and volume of red blood cells. Options (a), (b), and (d) may be manifested as a result of the rise in the number of red blood cells.___

3. The nurse is caring for a client scheduled for hemodialysis this morning. In preparing the client for the dialysis treatment, it is most important for the nurse to:
   a. allow the client to rest until after the dialysis treatment.
   b. ensure that all morning care is completed before dialysis.
   c. make the client NPO until after the dialysis treatment.
   d. withhold the morning dose of any antihypertensive drugs.

   Rationale: ___The answer is (d). Hypotension is a complication of dialysis. Antihypertensive drugs taken before dialysis can cause severe hypotension. Options (a) and (b) are not the most important in preparing the client, and option (c) is not necessary in preparing the client for hemodialysis.___

2-11 THE PATIENT WITH PERIPHERAL ARTERIAL DISEASE (DEVELOPMENT OF SIGNS AND SYMPTOMS OF GANGRENE)

Mr. L, 70 years old, is sent to the hospital after visiting his physician with complaints of increasing painful muscle cramps after ambulating. He lives alone and his medical history is significant for hypertension. The nursing care Kardex has the following admission orders:

VS q4h I & O (✓) Pedal pulse check q4h Bed rest with BRP CBC, UA, Electrolytes Mr. L Age: 70	Insert saline lock Drsg chgs: Clean ulcerated area on left lateral ankle with NS—apply dry sterile 4 × 4s Dx: Peripheral artery disease	Diet: mech soft Routine med: Pentoxifylline 400 mg po tid Dipyridamole 50 mg po tid

You are assigned to begin his admission. You note that he is alert but hard of hearing. He has a bandage around his left foot. He tells you he uses this to keep his shoe from rubbing his foot. He has another bandage over his left ankle.

Prioritize the five **nursing interventions** as you would do them to take care of Mr. L. Write a number in the box to identify the order of your interventions (#1 = first intervention, #2 = second intervention, etc.) and state a **rationale** for each intervention.

INTERVENTIONS	PRIORITY #	RATIONALE
• Take the VS, pulse ox, assess pain level	☐	_____
• Assess bilateral pedal pulses	☐	_____
• Orient to hospital room	☐	_____
• Perform a body systems assessment	☐	_____
• Apply sterile dressing to left ankle	☐	_____

KEY POINTS TO CONSIDER _____

_____

_____

_____

You assist Mr. L to the bathroom; on his return to bed you note the following:
1. Bilateral lower extremities—reddish blue in color.
2. Bilateral pedal pulses weak (1+), capillary refill greater than 3 seconds.
3. The skin of the lower extremities is cool, tight, and shiny.
4. Gait slow, needs assistance.

Integrated Learning Activity: With a partner, **do the following: (1) select** the **one nursing diagnosis** that is a priority at this time, **(2) provide a rationale** for your selection, and **(3) list the nursing interventions** that assist you to meet the needs of the patient.

All of the following nursing diagnoses may apply to Mr. L:

Risk for injury: fall, Deficient knowledge, Risk for infection, Impaired skin integrity, Impaired physical mobility, Ineffective peripheral tissue perfusion, Activity intolerance, Impaired tissue integrity, Acute pain

Nursing Diagnosis	Rationale	Nursing Interventions
Ineffective peripheral tissue perfusion	- LE blue, weak - LE cool, tight, shiny - pulses +1 (pedal) - cap. refill > 3 sec.	- ___ to bed - walks - ___

After having changed the dressing on the left ankle, you **remove the bandage** from the left foot and you note: two discolored shrunken black toes.

On the basis of **removal of the bandage** information, identify and write the **priority problem** in the box below. Then, starting with the small box labeled **#1, prioritize** the **nursing interventions** for this situation and **identify** your follow-up action plan for Mr. L.

NURSING INTERVENTIONS

A. Assess pain level

B. Measure blackened area

C. Put on sterile gloves

D. Cleanse area with normal saline solution

E. Apply sterile dressing

F. Document assessment findings

DECISION-MAKING DIAGRAM

New Action Plan

#1	#2	#3	#4	#5	#6
A	C	B	D	E	F

Priority Problem

infection, necrosis

NOTES _____

2-12 THE PATIENT WITH CHEST PAIN (DEVELOPMENT OF CHEST PAIN)

The handoff shift report includes: Mrs. T, 56 years old, was admitted around midnight from the ER after experiencing some chest pain. She has coronary artery disease and smokes one pack of cigarettes a day. Her father died of heart disease and she has a brother with hypertension. Her VS are T 98° F, P 90, R 26, BP 164/100, pain level 0, pulse ox 97%. Mrs. T has been taking verapamil, nifedipine, and atenolol. Mrs. T will continue with her usual cardiac and blood pressure medications and is also started on aspirin 81 mg, docusate sodium, and lovastatin. Nitroglycerin tablets 0.4 mg SL are ordered prn chest pain and has Mylanta 30 mL q2h prn. She has bathroom privileges with assistance, a saline lock, and oxygen at 3 L/min/nasal cannula to keep the oxygen saturation greater than 96%. Mrs. T is upset about not being able to get up and smoke. Mrs. T is requesting to use the commode as you start your shift.

Prioritize the five **nursing interventions** as you would do them to initially take care of Mrs. T. Write a number in the box to identify the order of your interventions (#1 = first intervention, #2 = second intervention, etc.) and state a **rationale** for each intervention.

INTERVENTIONS	PRIORITY #	RATIONALE
• Take the vital signs and assess pain level	☐	_____
• Assist to commode	☐	_____
• Perform a body systems assessment	☐	_____
• Check oxygen saturation level	☐	_____
• Talk with Mrs. T	☐	_____

KEY POINTS TO CONSIDER _____

_____

_____

After breakfast Mrs. T continues to be upset. She states that she is constipated and above all wants to smoke. She is getting increasingly upset. You observe the following:

1. Abdomen round, bowel sounds present in all four quadrants
2. Breakfast intake 30%
3. Last bowel movement 2 days ago
4. SOB, oxygen saturation at 93%

Integrated Learning Activity: With a partner, **do the following: (1) select** the **one nursing diagnosis** that is a priority at this time, **(2) provide a rationale** for your selection, and **(3) list the nursing interventions** that assist you to meet the needs of the patient.

All of the following nursing diagnoses may apply to Mrs. T:

Acute pain, Deficient knowledge, Anxiety, Noncompliance, Ineffective coping, Decreased cardiac output, Activity intolerance, Risk for impaired skin integrity, Constipation, Ineffective health maintenance

Nursing Diagnosis	Rationale	Nursing Interventions

At **10:00 AM** the nursing assistant reports that Mrs. T is feeling chest pain. You assess and note that she has cool, clammy skin, complains of indigestion and tightness in her chest. BP 154/98, P 100, R 30, states chest pain at a level of 8. Oxygen saturation is 88%.

On the basis of the data at **10:00 AM**, identify and write the **priority problem** in the box below. Then, starting with the small box labeled **#1, prioritize** the **nursing interventions** for this situation and **identify** your follow-up action plan for Mrs. T.

NURSING INTERVENTIONS   DECISION-MAKING DIAGRAM

A.   Oxygen @ 3 L/min/NC

B.   Activate the hospital's Rapid Response Team

C.   Administer nitroglycerin
     tab i q5min × 3

New Action Plan

     #1   #2   #3   #4   #5   #6

D.   Monitor VS q5min

E.   Obtain 12-lead electro-
     cardiogram per protocol

F.   Notify physician

NOTES _____

Priority Problem _____

2-13 THE PATIENT WITH HEART FAILURE (DEVELOPMENT OF CARDIAC ARREST)

You are assigned to Mr. T who was transferred to your unit earlier today. In the handoff report you learn that he has heart failure (HF), 3+ pitting edema of the lower extremities, and increasing shortness of breath. He has been demonstrating Cheyne-Stokes respirations and periods of confusion and complains of blurred vision. Vital signs are T 97.6° F, P 62, R 22, BP 180/102, pain level 0, pulse ox 96%. He has received his 0900 meds. Current orders include:

VS q4h. I & O (✓) Up in chair qid O$_2$ @ 3 L/min/NP Serum K$^+$, PT, PTT, ABG (✓) Chest x-ray (✓) ECG (✓) Name: T. Age: 72	IV D5W @ 50 mL/hr IV site: LFA #20 g LBM: 2 days ago Foley (✓) Code Status: Full code Dx: Heart failure	Diet: Soft (NAS) Routine medications: Digoxin 0.25 mg IVP qAM 0900 Furosemide 40 mg po bid 0900-1700 Docusate sodium 100 mg tab i po qAM 0900 Prazosin 10 mg po bid 0900-1700

Prioritize the five **nursing interventions** as you would do them to take care of Mr. T. Write a number in the box to identify the order of your interventions (#1 = first intervention, #2 = second intervention, etc.) and state a **rationale** for each intervention.

INTERVENTIONS	PRIORITY #	RATIONALE
• Assess respiratory rate	☐	_____ _____
• Obtain urinary output data	☐	_____ _____
• Assess rate/rhythm and quality of pulse	☐	_____ _____
• Assess complaints of visual disturbances	☐	_____ _____
• Check current lab data	☐	_____ _____

KEY POINTS TO CONSIDER _____

_____

_____

_____

Mr. T wants to wash up, but he says that he does not have the energy like he used to and that he gets tired very easily. You assist him with morning care and assess the following:

1. Skin cool, dusky in color
2. Lower extremities with 2+ pitting edema
3. Lung sounds with crackles on inspiration; R 24, regular pattern
4. Alert and oriented at this time

Integrated Learning Activity: With a partner, **do the following: (1) select** the **one nursing diagnosis** that is a priority at this time, **(2) provide a rationale** for your selection, and **(3) list the nursing interventions** that assist you to meet the needs of the patient.

All of the following nursing diagnoses may apply to Mr. T:

Anxiety, Risk for infection, Activity intolerance, Excess fluid volume, Impaired tissue integrity, Risk for ineffective cerebral tissue perfusion, Imbalanced nutrition: less than body requirements, Risk for injury, Deficient knowledge, Impaired gas exchange, Fatigue

Nursing Diagnosis	Rationale	Nursing Interventions

Mr. T's family stops to visit during lunch. **At 1:00 PM,** the nursing assistant tells you that Mr. T is in distress. You walk into the room and notice Mr. T holding his chest tightly. Shortly afterward you assess: cyanosis, no pulse, no BP, and no respirations.

On the basis of the situation at **1:00 PM,** identify and write the **priority problem** in the box below. Then, starting with the small box labeled **#1, prioritize** the **nursing interventions** for this situation and **identify** your follow-up action plan for Mr. T.

NURSING INTERVENTIONS   **DECISION-MAKING DIAGRAM**

A. Call the Code Team/Rapid Response Team

B. Place in supine position

C. Begin CPR

D. Notify physician

E. Document findings

F. Support family

New Action Plan

#1 #2 #3 #4 #5 #6

Priority Problem

NOTES _____

_____

APPLYING CRITICAL THINKING SKILLS TO TEST QUESTIONS

INSTRUCTIONS: Circle the one best answer for each test question. Write your rationale for selecting the answer. To enhance your learning and test-taking skills, discuss your answer and rationale with a partner. The answer and the rationale can be found on the back of this page.

1. The nurse admits a 69-year-old male client with heart failure. The physician orders furosemide 60 mg IVP stat, digoxin 0.25 mg po, and KCl 20 mEq po now. Which assessment finding is most indicative of an ineffective response 2 hours after the administration of all the medications?
   a. Pulse 89, irregular
   b. Urine output 60 mL
   c. Pulse oximetry 94%
   d. Pitting edema in the lower extremities

   Rationale: _____
   _____
   _____
   _____
   _____

2. The home health nurse visits a client with heart failure. In reviewing the client's medications, the nurse notes that the client takes the following daily oral medications: digoxin 0.25 mg, furosemide 10 mg, and captopril 0.625 mg. After speaking to the client and wife, the nurse suspects digitalis toxicity. Which question helps the nurse gather more information specific to digitalis toxicity?
   a. "Do you get light-headed when you get out of bed?"
   b. "Do you need to sleep with more than one pillow?"
   c. "Do you have to get up to urinate more frequently?"
   d. "Have you had any nausea, vomiting, or diarrhea?"

   Rationale: _____
   _____
   _____
   _____
   _____

3. The nurse is assigned to a client with heart failure. The nurse's morning lung assessment indicates crackles and wheezes in the mid to lower lung bases, R 32, and the client is restless. Which nursing intervention is of priority initially?
   a. Assess capillary refill
   b. Take the pulse oximetry
   c. Limit client activity
   d. Assess fluid intake

   Rationale: _____
   _____
   _____
   _____
   _____

ANSWER KEY FOR
APPLYING CRITICAL THINKING SKILLS TO TEST QUESTIONS

HELPFUL HINTS: Read all test questions carefully. Identify key words in the question that will guide you in answering the question. In these test questions the **key words** to consider are **"most indicative," "specific information,"** and **"priority initially."** Compare your rationale with the one in the test question.

1. The nurse admits a 69-year-old male client with heart failure. The physician orders furosemide 60 mg IVP stat, digoxin 0.25 mg po, and KCl 20 mEq po now. Which assessment finding is most indicative of an ineffective response 2 hours after the administration of all the medications?
   a. Pulse 89, irregular
   b. Urine output 60 mL
   c. Pulse oximetry 94%
   d. Pitting edema in the lower extremities

   Rationale: ___The answer is (b). Although output falls within the parameters of renal function, the client received furosemide IV and diuresis is the desired effect. Options (a), (c), and (d) are expected findings in a client with HF.___

2. The home health nurse visits a client with heart failure. In reviewing the client's medications, the nurse notes that the client takes the following daily oral medications: digoxin 0.25 mg, furosemide 10 mg, and captopril 0.625 mg. After speaking to the client and wife, the nurse suspects digitalis toxicity. Which question helps the nurse gather more information specific to digitalis toxicity?
   a. "Do you get light-headed when you get out of bed?"
   b. "Do you need to sleep with more than one pillow?"
   c. "Do you have to get up to urinate more frequently?"
   d. "Have you had any nausea, vomiting, or diarrhea?"

   Rationale: ___The answer is (d). Although these signs and symptoms are frequently seen with all drug therapy, they are frequently early side effects of digitalis toxicity. Options (a), (b), and (c) relate to the action of the other drugs.___

3. The nurse is assigned to a client with heart failure. The nurse's morning lung assessment indicates crackles and wheezes in the mid to lower lung bases, R 32, and the client is restless. Which nursing intervention is of priority initially?
   a. Assess capillary refill
   b. Take the pulse oximetry
   c. Limit client activity
   d. Assess fluid intake

   Rationale: ___The answer is (b). Client assessment indicates rapid breathing and possible hypoxia. To fully assess the respiratory status of the client, it is important to take the pulse oximetry. Options (a), (c), and (d) are important—but not priority—interventions.___

2-14 THE PATIENT WITH A STROKE (DEVELOPMENT OF ADVERSE EFFECTS—HEPARIN THERAPY)

Mr. H, 68 years old, has had a right-sided stroke. He was admitted to the telemetry unit 2 days ago and he has been on heparin therapy. The latest documentation in the nursing notes shows: Hand grips R stronger than L, speech slurred, BP 166/102. The orders in the nursing care Kardex include the following:

VS q4h   I & O (✔)
Neuro checks q4h
Up in chair today
 	
O₂ @ 2 L/min/NP
 	
Hospital day: #3
	IV: 500 mL: D5W with heparin 10,000 units infuse at 1000 units/hr
	
	Foley (✔) care bid
	ROM to left upper and lower extremities
	
	Serum K⁺, Na⁺ & CBC today
	PTT daily
		Diet: Dysphagia (to be determined after swallow evaluation)
		
		Swallowing precautions
		
		Routine med:
		  Docusate sodium 20 mg (5 mL) po
		    bid
		  Nimodipine 20 mg po tid

You begin your shift and during the handoff report you learn that Mr. H had a restful night and there were no changes in his condition. You prepare to assist Mr. H with his breakfast.

Prioritize the five **nursing interventions** as you would do them to take care of Mr. H. Write a number in the box to identify the order of your interventions (#1 = first intervention, #2 = second intervention, etc.) and state a **rationale** for each intervention.

INTERVENTIONS	PRIORITY #	RATIONALE
• Sit in Fowler position	☐	_____ _____
• Place food on right side for patient to see	☐	_____ _____
• Place food into stronger side of mouth	☐	_____ _____
• Check inside of mouth for food caught between gums and teeth (pocketing)	☐	_____ _____
• Maintain Fowler position for 30-45 minutes	☐	_____ _____

KEY POINTS TO CONSIDER _____
_____
_____
_____

As morning care is given to Mr. H you assess the following:
1. Does not turn head if spoken to from left side
2. Left hand and arm elevated on a pillow
3. Passive range of motion is performed to extremities on the left side
4. Antiembolic stockings on with sequential compression device on
5. Lack of awareness of left side

Integrated Learning Activity: With a partner, **do the following: (1) select** the **one nursing diagnosis** that is a priority at this time, **(2) provide a rationale** for your selection, and **(3) list the nursing interventions** that assist you to meet the needs of the patient.

All of the following nursing diagnoses may apply to Mr. H:

Risk for injury: falls, Deficient knowledge, Fear, Anxiety, Risk for infection, Impaired tissue integrity, Constipation, Impaired swallowing, Impaired verbal communication, Bathing self-care deficit, Impaired urinary elimination, Disturbed body image, Risk for impaired skin integrity, Ineffective peripheral tissue perfusion, Unilateral neglect, Risk for aspiration, Risk for disuse syndrome

Nursing Diagnosis	Rationale	Nursing Interventions

Mr. H's laboratory data are called to the unit. The results are as follows: PTT 250 sec (control 38 sec), K^+ 3.5 mEq, Na^+ 145 mEq, Hgb 11.4 g/dL, Hct 34%, platelets 110,000/mm^3

Based on **Mr. H's laboratory** data, identify and write the **priority problem** in the box below. Then, starting with the small box labeled **#1, prioritize** the **nursing interventions** for this situation and **identify** your follow-up action plan for Mr. H.

NURSING INTERVENTIONS

A. Notify physician

B. Prepare to administer protamine sulfate (if ordered)

C. Assess for petechiae

D. Monitor urine color

E. Monitor neuro status

F. Take the VS

DECISION-MAKING DIAGRAM

New Action Plan

#1 #2 #3 #4 #5 #6

☐ ☐ ☐ ☐ ☐ ☐

Priority Problem

NOTES _____

_____

APPLYING CRITICAL THINKING SKILLS TO TEST QUESTIONS

INSTRUCTIONS: Circle the one best answer for each test question. Write your rationale for selecting the answer. To enhance your learning and test-taking skills, discuss your answer and rationale with a partner. The answer and the rationale can be found on the back of this page.

1. The nurse is caring for a client who had a right-sided stroke 5 days ago and is experiencing unilateral neglect. In delegating the care of the client, which nursing intervention is of priority? The nurse instructs the nursing assistant to:
   a. have the client use a communication board.
   b. place the food tray to the right side of the body.
   c. remind the client to look at the left side of the body.
   d. provide passive range of motion to the left side of the body.

   Rationale: _____
   _____
   _____
   _____
   _____

2. The nurse walks into a client's room. The client is in supine position and the wife is stroking his hand. The client had a left-sided stroke 7 days ago, just took 30% of the dysphagic diet, and has an indwelling urinary catheter. Which nursing action is of priority for this client?
   a. Raise the head of the bed.
   b. Encourage the wife to talk softly to the client.
   c. Remind the client to look and touch the affected side.
   d. Assess the color and amount of output.

   Rationale: _____
   _____
   _____
   _____
   _____

3. The nurse is preparing to administer oral medications to a client who is on a dysphagic diet. Which nursing action is best in administering the 0900 medication to the client? Crush the medication and:
   a. put the crushed medication in 15 mL of tap water.
   b. mix the crushed medication in 4 ounces of applesauce.
   c. dissolve the crushed medication in 30 mL of warm water.
   d. mix the crushed medication in 30 mL of thickened liquid.

   Rationale: _____
   _____
   _____
   _____
   _____

ANSWER KEY FOR
APPLYING CRITICAL THINKING SKILLS TO TEST QUESTIONS

HELPFUL HINTS: Read all test questions carefully. Identify key words in the question that will guide you in answering the question. In these test questions the **key words** to consider are **"priority"** and **"best."** Compare your rationale with the one in the test question.

1. The nurse is caring for a client who had a right-sided stroke 5 days ago and is experiencing unilateral neglect. In delegating the care of the client, which nursing intervention is of priority? The nurse instructs the nursing assistant to:
   a. have the client use a communication board.
   b. place the food tray to the right side of the body.
   c. remind the client to look at the left side of the body.
   d. provide passive range of motion to the left side of the body.

   Rationale: The answer is (c). Clients who have a right-sided stroke have spatial and perceptual deficits. Clients will neglect the left side of the body. Options (a), (b), and (d) do not correlate the clients need to the intervention.

2. The nurse walks into a client's room. The client is in supine position and the wife is stroking his hand. The client had a left-sided stroke 7 days ago, just took 30% of the dysphagic diet, and has an indwelling urinary catheter. Which nursing action is of priority for this client?
   a. Raise the head of the bed.
   b. Encourage the wife to talk softly to the client.
   c. Remind the client to look and touch the affected side.
   d. Assess the color and amount of output.

   Rationale: The answer is (a). After eating, the client should remain in Fowler position to prevent aspiration. Options (b), (c), and (d) are important, but they are not priorities at this time.

3. The nurse is preparing to administer oral medications to a client who is on a dysphagic diet. Which nursing action is best in administering the 0900 medication to the client? Crush the medication and:
   a. put the crushed medication in 15 mL of tap water.
   b. mix the crushed medication in 4 ounces of applesauce.
   c. dissolve the crushed medication in 30 mL of warm water.
   d. mix the crushed medication in 30 mL of thickened liquid.

   Rationale: The answer is (d). Use a small amount of thickened liquids to mix and administer the medications. Options (a) and (c) are not appropriate because water may cause the client to aspirate. Option (b) is mixing the medications in too large a quantity of applesauce.

2-15 THE PATIENT WITH CHRONIC OBSTRUCTIVE PULMONARY DISEASE (DEVELOPMENT OF SIGNS AND SYMPTOMS OF RESPIRATORY INFECTION)

TWO

You are assigned to Mr. Y, a 66-year-old man who has chronic obstructive pulmonary disease (COPD). In the handoff morning report you learn that he has been agitated during the night and is dyspneic this morning. The 0600 vital signs are T 98.8° F, P 102, R 32, BP 146/98, denies pain. His 0700 pulse oximeter reading was 89% (room air) and he has an aminophylline drip infusing at 6 mg/hr per pump and oxygen at 2 L/min/nasal cannula. He receives albuterol inhaler 2 puffs q4h and ipratropium (Atrovent) inhaler 2 puffs q4h. He had a serum theophylline level drawn in the evening. It is now 0730.

Prioritize the five **nursing interventions** as you would do them to initially take care of Mr. Y. Write a number in the box to identify the order of your interventions (#1 = first intervention, #2 = second intervention, etc.) and state a **rationale** for each intervention.

INTERVENTIONS	PRIORITY #	RATIONALE
• Auscultate lung sounds	☐	_____
• Assess pulse oximeter, oxygen, and nasal cannula	☐	_____
• Retake the vital signs	☐	_____
• Check theophylline level	☐	_____
• Place in high Fowler position	☐	_____

KEY POINTS TO CONSIDER _____

As you provide morning care to Mr. Y you note the following signs and symptoms:
1. Nonproductive cough; long expiratory phase during respiration
2. Increased shortness of breath with mild exertion
3. Crackles audible throughout the bilateral lung fields
4. Anxious and restless
5. Theophylline level 14 mcg/mL

⚡ **Integrated Learning Activity:** With a partner, **do the following: (1) select** the **one nursing diagnosis** that is a priority at this time, **(2) provide a rationale** for your selection, and **(3) list the nursing interventions** that assist you to meet the needs of the patient.

All of the following nursing diagnoses may apply to Mr. Y:

Ineffective breathing pattern, Ineffective airway clearance, Risk for injury, Risk for infection, Anxiety, Impaired gas exchange, Activity intolerance, Risk for impaired skin integrity, Imbalanced nutrition: less than body requirements, Sexual dysfunction

Nursing Diagnosis	Rationale	Nursing Interventions

At **12:00 noon** the patient care assistant reports that Mr. Y is very warm and that his VS are T 102° F, P 98, R 32, BP 140/84. He is expectorating thick yellow-colored sputum.

Based on the situation at **12:00 noon,** identify and write the **priority problem** in the box below. Then, starting with the small box labeled **#1, prioritize** the **nursing interventions** for this situation and **identify** your follow-up action plan for Mr. Y.

NURSING INTERVENTIONS   DECISION-MAKING DIAGRAM

A. Auscultate lung sounds

B. Administer antipyretic if ordered

C. Assess orientation and LOC

D. Check oxygen saturation level

E. Retake VS in 2 hr

F. Inform physician

New Action Plan

#1   #2   #3   #4   #5   #6

Priority Problem

NOTES _____

_____

APPLYING CRITICAL THINKING SKILLS TO TEST QUESTIONS

INSTRUCTIONS: Circle the one best answer for each test question. Write your rationale for selecting the answer. To enhance your learning and test-taking skills, discuss your answer and rationale with a partner. The answer and the rationale can be found on the back of this page.

1. The nurse is caring for a client who was admitted with an exacerbation of COPD. The client's respirations are 28 with dyspnea on exertion. The client is receiving 2 L of oxygen per nasal cannula. The morning pulse oximetry is 92%. Which nursing intervention is of priority?
   a. Monitor the client.
   b. Notify the physician.
   c. Get an order to increase the oxygen.
   d. Place in semi-Fowler position.

   Rationale: _____
   _____
   _____
   _____
   _____

2. The client has a long history of COPD and is currently experiencing an exacerbation of COPD. The following lab work is done this morning: complete blood cell count, arterial blood gases, and an electrolyte panel consisting of K^+, Na^+, Cl^-, carbon dioxide, blood urea nitrogen, and fasting blood glucose. Which laboratory data will require immediate follow-up?
   a. PaO_2 WNL
   b. Increased RBCs
   c. Increased $PaCO_2$
   d. Hgb WNL

   Rationale: _____
   _____
   _____
   _____
   _____

3. The client is admitted with an acute exacerbation of COPD. Which assessment finding is most indicative of a potential complication?
   a. R 32, increasingly anxious and restless
   b. Using accessory muscles during respiration
   c. Pulse oximetry 92%, purse-lip breathing
   d. Expectorating copious amount of white phlegm

   Rationale: _____
   _____
   _____
   _____
   _____

ANSWER KEY FOR
APPLYING CRITICAL THINKING SKILLS TO TEST QUESTIONS

HELPFUL HINTS: Read all test questions carefully. Identify key words in the question that will guide you in answering the question. In these test questions the **key words** to consider are **"priority," "immediate,"** and **"most indicative."** Compare your rationale with the one in the test question.

1. The nurse is caring for a client who was admitted with an exacerbation of COPD. The client's respirations are 28 with dyspnea on exertion. The client is receiving 2 L of oxygen per nasal cannula. The morning pulse oximetry is 92%. Which nursing intervention is of priority?
   a. Monitor the client.
   b. Notify the physician.
   c. Get an order to increase the oxygen.
   d. Place in semi-Fowler position.

   Rationale: The answer is (a). The client is manifesting signs and symptoms consistent with COPD. Clients with COPD have some degree of hypoxia. Options (b) and (c) are not appropriate at this time. Option (d) is not the best position for a client with COPD.

2. The client has a long history of COPD and is currently experiencing an exacerbation of COPD. The following lab work is done this morning: complete blood cell count, arterial blood gases, and an electrolyte panel consisting of K^+, Na^+, Cl^-, carbon dioxide, blood urea nitrogen, and fasting blood glucose. Which laboratory data will require immediate follow-up?
   a. PaO_2 WNL
   b. Increased RBCs
   c. Increased $PaCO_2$
   d. Hgb WNL

   Rationale: The answer is (a). Hypoxemia provides the stimulus for the respiratory drive in client with COPD. Increased oxygen levels may depress the respiratory drive. Options (b) and (c) are expected findings. Option (d) does not require immediate follow-up.

3. The client is admitted with an acute exacerbation of COPD. Which assessment finding is most indicative of a potential complication?
   a. R 32, increasingly anxious and restless
   b. Using accessory muscles during respiration
   c. Pulse oximetry 92%, purse-lip breathing
   d. Expectorating copious amount of white phlegm

   Rationale: The answer is (a). Increasing anxiousness and restlessness are signs indicating hypoxemia. Options (b), (c), (d) are expected findings for a client with an exacerbation of COPD.

2-16 THE PATIENT WITH A CHEST TUBE (DEVELOPMENT OF SIGNS AND SYMPTOMS OF RESPIRATORY INSUFFICIENCY)

Mr. G, 23 years old, has been in the hospital for 2 days after being stabbed in the chest. He has a posterior chest tube connected to a Pleur-Evac system. You are assigned to his care and the nursing care Kardex contains the following information:

VS q4h I & O (✓) Pulse ox q4h Amb with assist prn O_2 @ 2-3 L/min/NP Chest tube to low con't suction	IV: D5/0.45 NS q12h IVPB: cefazolin 1 g q6h Chest x-ray today ABG today	Diet: Soft Routine med: Colace 100 mg po daily

The 7:00 AM handoff report indicates that he had a restful night. Pain level 2. Chest tube drainage was 15 mL. Midnight VS were T 99° F, P 90, R 22, BP 128/74. Pulse ox at 4:00 AM was 95%, O_2 @ 3 L/min/NP.

Prioritize the five **nursing interventions** as you would do them to take care of Mr. G. Write a number in the box to identify the order of your interventions (#1 = first intervention, #2 = second intervention, etc.) and state a **rationale** for each intervention.

INTERVENTIONS	PRIORITY #	RATIONALE
• Check the pulse oximetry	☐	_____
• Assess for fluctuation in the water-seal chamber and bubbling in the suction-control chamber	☐	_____
• Check for the previous shift's fluid level marking on the tape	☐	_____
• Assess chest tube patency and drainage	☐	_____
• Ask Mr. G to cough and deep breathe	☐	_____

KEY POINTS TO CONSIDER _____

After breakfast, Mr. G is transported to the x-ray department by wheelchair. On his return to his room you assess the following:

1. VS: T 99.8° F, P 102, R 26, BP 132/90
2. Complains of dyspnea, crackles auscultated, anxious
3. Oxygen off, oxygen saturation at 88%

⚡**Integrated Learning Activity:** With a partner, **do the following: (1) select** the **one nursing diagnosis** that is a priority at this time, **(2) provide a rationale** for your selection, and **(3) list the nursing interventions** that assist you to meet the needs of the patient.

All of the following nursing diagnoses may apply to Mr. G:

Ineffective airway clearance, Ineffective breathing pattern, Impaired gas exchange, Risk for injury, Deficient knowledge, Fear, Anxiety, Risk for infection, Impaired tissue integrity

Nursing Diagnosis	Rationale	Nursing Interventions

One hour later, Mr. G becomes increasingly restless and, as you take his VS, he abruptly moves and the chest tube is pulled out.

On the basis of the situation **1 hour later,** identify and write the **priority problem** in the box below. Then, starting with the small box labeled **#1, prioritize** the **nursing interventions** for this situation and **identify** your follow-up action plan for Mr. G.

NURSING INTERVENTIONS   DECISION-MAKING DIAGRAM

A. Instruct Mr. G to take a deep breath and hold

B. Cover chest tube site with occlusive dressing

C. Apply gloves if possible

D. Maintain oxygen @ 3 L/min/NP

E. Notify physician

F. Pinch chest tube site together

New Action Plan

#1   #2   #3   #4   #5   #6

□   □   □   □   □   □

Priority Problem

NOTES _____

_____

APPLYING CRITICAL THINKING SKILLS TO TEST QUESTIONS

INSTRUCTIONS: Circle the one best answer for each test question. Write your rationale for selecting the answer. To enhance your learning and test-taking skills, discuss your answer and rationale with a partner. The answer and the rationale can be found on the back of this page.

1. The nurse is preparing to assist with the insertion of a chest tube that will be attached to a closed-chest drainage system without suction. In monitoring the closed-chest drainage system, the nurse would expect to initially assess for:
   a. fluctuation of water in the water-seal chamber during respirations.
   b. constant fluid fluctuations in the drainage-collection chamber.
   c. continuous bubbling in the suction-control chamber.
   d. occasional bubbling in the suction-control chamber.

   Rationale: _____
   _____
   _____
   _____
   _____

2. The client has a chest tube connected to a closed-chest drainage system attached to suction and is being prepared to transfer to another room on a stretcher. To safely transport the client, it is most important for the nurse to:
   a. clamp the chest tube during the transport.
   b. get a portable suction before transferring the client.
   c. keep the closed-chest drainage system below the level of the chest.
   d. place the closed-chest drainage system next to the client on the stretcher.

   Rationale: _____
   _____
   _____
   _____
   _____

3. The physician is preparing to remove the client's chest tube. Just before removing the chest tube, the physician tells the client to take a deep breath and hold it. The intervention is primarily done to:
   a. distract the client during the chest tube removal.
   b. minimize the negative pressure within the pleural space.
   c. decrease the degree of discomfort to the client.
   d. increase the intrathoracic pressure temporarily during removal.

   Rationale: _____
   _____
   _____
   _____
   _____

ANSWER KEY FOR
APPLYING CRITICAL THINKING SKILLS TO TEST QUESTIONS

HELPFUL HINTS: Read all test questions carefully. Identify key words in the question that will guide you in answering the question. In these test questions the **key words** to consider are **"initially," "most important,"** and **"primarily."** Compare your rationale with the one in the test question.

1. The nurse is preparing to assist with the insertion of a chest tube that will be attached to a closed-chest drainage system without suction. In monitoring the closed-chest drainage system, the nurse would expect to initially assess for:
   a. fluctuation of water in the water-seal chamber during respirations.
   b. constant fluid fluctuations in the drainage-collection chamber.
   c. continuous bubbling in the suction-control chamber.
   d. occasional bubbling in the suction-control chamber.

   Rationale: _The answer is (a). Fluctuations of water during inspiration and expiration in the water-seal chamber indicates normal functioning. Option (b) should not be seen in the collection chamber. Options (c) and (d) should not be seen because suction has not been applied to the suction-control chamber._

2. The client has a chest tube connected to a closed-chest drainage system attached to suction and is being prepared to transfer to another room on a stretcher. To safely transport the client, it is most important for the nurse to:
   a. clamp the chest tube during the transport.
   b. get a portable suction before transferring the client.
   c. keep the closed-chest drainage system below the level of the chest.
   d. place the closed-chest drainage system next to the client on the stretcher.

   Rationale: _The answer is (c). Keeping the closed-chest drainage system below the level of the chest allows for continuous drainage and prevents any backflow pressure. Options (a) and (d) should not be done because they will increase pressure in the pleural space. Option (b) is not the most important._

3. The physician is preparing to remove the client's chest tube. Just before removing the chest tube, the physician tells the client to take a deep breath and hold it. The intervention is primarily done to:
   a. distract the client during the chest tube removal.
   b. minimize the negative pressure within the pleural space.
   c. decrease the degree of discomfort to the client.
   d. increase the intrathoracic pressure temporarily during removal.

   Rationale: _The answer is (d). This is done to decrease the risk of atmospheric air entering the pleural space during removal. Options (a) and (c) are not the primary reasons for this intervention. Option (b) is not correct because negative pressure is desired within the lung._

2-17 THE PATIENT WITH UROSEPSIS (DEVELOPMENT OF SIGNS AND SYMPTOMS OF SEPTIC SHOCK)

Mr. TD, 79 years old, was admitted today to the hospital with the diagnosis of urosepsis. He has an IV of lactated Ringer's infusing at 100 mL/hr. Ceftriaxone 1 g IVPB qAM is ordered. He is on I & O q8h, soft diet, bathroom privileges with assistance and acetaminophen 500 mg tabs i po q4h for temperature greater than 38° C. The day shift handoff report indicated his VS were T 38° C, P 78, R 22, BP 146/88, pulse ox 96% at 2:00 PM. The nurse also said that he was more restless this afternoon and had been trying to get out of bed and seemed somewhat disoriented. He did not receive acetaminophen, but he was moved closer to the nurse's station to assist with frequent monitoring. You have been assigned as his nurse for the evening shift.

Prioritize the following **nursing interventions** as you, the nurse, would do them to initially take care of Mr. TD. Write a number in the box to identify the order of your interventions (#1 = first intervention, #2 = second intervention, etc.) and state a **rationale** for each intervention.

INTERVENTIONS	PRIORITY #	RATIONALE
• Assess for bed alarm/safety features	☐	_____
• Take VS	☐	_____
• Gather urinary output data	☐	_____
• Assess mental status	☐	_____
• Perform a body systems physical assessment	☐	_____

KEY POINTS TO CONSIDER _____

_____

_____

TWO

You perform a follow-up assessment at 7:00 PM and note the following:
1. VS: T 38.5° C, P 98, R 22, BP 120/76, pulse ox 94%
2. Fine crackles audible on auscultation in the bilateral lower lung fields
3. He is sleepy, lethargic
4. He was incontinent of a scant amount of urine

✍ **Integrated Learning Activity:** With a partner, **do the following: (1) select** the **one nursing diagnosis** that is a priority at this time, **(2) provide a rationale** for your selection, and **(3) list the nursing interventions** that assist you to meet the needs of the patient.

All of the following nursing diagnoses may apply to Mr. TD:

Risk for impaired skin integrity, Impaired urinary elimination, Risk for injury, Acute confusion, Hyperthermia, Deficient fluid volume, Imbalanced nutrition: less than body requirements, Risk for shock, Ineffective breathing pattern, Fatigue

Nursing Diagnosis	Rationale	Nursing Interventions

As you take his **8:00 PM** vital signs, you note the following signs and symptoms: Lethargic, skin very warm and flushed, VS: T 39.1° C, P 130, R 28, BP 90/54, pulse ox 88%.

Based on the situation at **8:00 PM,** identify and write the **priority problem** in the box below. Then, starting with the small box labeled **#1, prioritize** the **nursing interventions** for this situation and **identify** your follow-up action plan for Mr. TD.

NURSING INTERVENTIONS   DECISION-MAKING DIAGRAM

A. Check pulse ox: attach probe to ear, nose, or forehead preferably

B. Prepare to start O$_2$

C. Prepare to insert indwelling urinary catheter

D. Take vital signs q5min

E. Document findings

F. Notify physician

New Action Plan

#1   #2   #3   #4   #5   #6

☐   ☐   ☐   ☐   ☐   ☐

NOTES _____

Priority Problem

_____

2-18 THE PATIENT WITH A TRANSURETHRAL RESECTION OF THE PROSTATE (DEVELOPMENT OF URINARY OBSTRUCTION)

Mr. J, 68 years old, had a TURP this morning after having been diagnosed with benign prostatic hypertrophy. Latest VS: T 98.2° F, P 88, R 20, BP 150/88 pulse ox 98%. The following postop orders have been noted:

VS q4h I & O – qs Antiembolic hose Sequential teds × 24 hr Up in chair this PM	IV: lactated Ringer's @100 mL/hr IV site: RFA # 20 g 3-way urinary catheter to gravity with continuous irrigation of NS to keep UA free of clots	Diet: Clear liquids this PM PRN medication: B & O supp. q4h prn bladder spasms

As you enter his room, Mr. J is alert, you notice that his urinary drainage bag is almost full with dark red urine and some blood clots; the normal saline solution irrigation bag is empty.

Prioritize the five **nursing interventions** as you would do them to take care of Mr. J. Write a number in the box to identify the order of your interventions (#1 = first intervention, #2 = second intervention, etc.) and state a **rationale** for each intervention.

INTERVENTIONS	PRIORITY #	RATIONALE
• Take VS, assess pain level	☐	_____
• Assess continuous urinary irrigation system	☐	_____
• Empty urinary drainage bag	☐	_____
• Perform a body systems physical assessment	☐	_____
• Hang up new normal saline solution irrigation bag	☐	_____

KEY POINTS TO CONSIDER _____

TWO

On the first postop day you assess the following on Mr. J:
1. VS: T 99.6° F, P 98, R 24, BP 154/90
2. Urinary catheter taped to thigh, urine pinkish, no clots
3. Grimaces and says, "I didn't think it would be this tough." States pain level 8 out of 10.
4. Further states, "I do not think sex will ever be the same."

Integrated Learning Activity: With a partner, **do the following: (1) select** the **one nursing diagnosis** that is a priority at this time, **(2) provide a rationale** for your selection, and **(3) list the nursing interventions** that assist you to meet the needs of the patient.

All of the following nursing diagnoses may apply to Mr. J:

Risk for infection, Impaired tissue integrity, Excess fluid volume, Deficient knowledge, Anxiety, Risk for injury, Impaired urinary elimination, Acute pain, Ineffective sexuality pattern, Situational low self-esteem, Urinary retention; Risk for bleeding

Nursing Diagnosis	Rationale	Nursing Interventions

The normal saline solution irrigation is discontinued at 12:00 noon the first postop day. Toward the end of the shift **(3:00 PM),** you **assess** the following on Mr. J: complaints of pain, states pain level 10, no output since 12:00 PM, abdominal distention, and Mr. J somewhat restless.

On the basis of the **3:00 PM assessment,** identify and write the **priority problem** in the box below. Then, starting with the small box labeled **#1,** prioritize the **nursing interventions** for this situation and **identify** your follow-up action plan for Mr. J.

NURSING INTERVENTIONS

A. Take the vital signs

B. Inform MD

C. Prepare to do a urinary irrigation

D. Give an antispasmodic

E. Place in low Fowler to semi-Fowler position

F. Encourage fluids

DECISION-MAKING DIAGRAM

New Action Plan

#1 #2 #3 #4 #5 #6

Priority Problem

NOTES _____

_____

APPLYING CRITICAL THINKING SKILLS TO TEST QUESTIONS

INSTRUCTIONS: Circle the one best answer for each test question. Write your rationale for selecting the answer. To enhance your learning and test-taking skills, discuss your answer and rationale with a partner. The answer and the rationale can be found on the back of this page.

1. The client is 1 day postop TURP. He has a three-way indwelling urinary catheter with continuous bladder irrigation. During handoff report, the nurse learns that the client's output was 1700 mL. A priority nursing intervention is for the nurse to:
   a. check the client's oral and parenteral intake for the previous shift.
   b. know the amount of irrigation fluid that infused during the previous shift.
   c. assess if the client has passed any urinary clots through the catheter.
   d. ensure that the urinary output is yellow to pinkish in color.

   Rationale: _____
   _____
   _____
   _____
   _____

2. The physician orders continuous bladder irrigation for a client who had a TURP this morning. To effectively implement this order, it is most important for the nurse to infuse the irrigation solution:
   a. to maintain urine output clear to light pink in color.
   b. when the urine is red with visible clots.
   c. so that the intake equals the output.
   d. at a rate of 50 mL/hr.

   Rationale: _____
   _____
   _____
   _____
   _____

3. The client is 2 days postop TURP and is complaining of an increasing urge to void. The client has a three-way urinary catheter with continuous bladder irrigation. After assessing that the catheter is patent and is draining freely, the priority nursing intervention is to:
   a. reassure the client that the catheter is draining appropriately.
   b. document the client's complaints and assessment findings.
   c. give the client antispasmodic medication.
   d. notify the physician.

   Rationale: _____
   _____
   _____
   _____
   _____

ANSWER KEY FOR
APPLYING CRITICAL THINKING SKILLS TO TEST QUESTIONS

HELPFUL HINTS: Read all test questions carefully. Identify key words in the question that will guide you in answering the question. In these test questions the **key words** to consider are **"priority"** and **"most important."** Compare your rationale with the one in the test question.

1. The client is 1 day postop TURP. He has a three-way indwelling urinary catheter with continuous bladder irrigation. During handoff report, the nurse learns that the client's output was 1700 mL. A priority nursing intervention is for the nurse to:
   a. check the client's oral and parenteral intake for the previous shift.
   b. know the amount of irrigation fluid that infused during the previous shift.
   c. assess if the client has passed any urinary clots through the catheter.
   d. ensure that the urinary output is yellow to pinkish in color.

   Rationale: ___The answer is (b). It is important to know the amount of irrigation solution that infused to assess the actual urinary output. Options (a), (c), and (d) are good interventions but not of priority.___

2. The physician orders continuous bladder irrigation for a client who had a TURP this morning. To effectively implement this order, it is most important for the nurse to infuse the irrigation solution:
   a. to maintain urine output clear to light pink in color.
   b. when the urine is red with visible clots.
   c. so that the intake equals the output.
   d. at a rate of 50 mL/hr.

   Rationale: ___The answer is (a). Continuous irrigation is given to prevent clot formation and prevent obstruction of the catheter. Options (b), (c), and (d) are not appropriate interventions.___

3. The client is 2 days postop TURP and is complaining of an increasing urge to void. The client has a three-way urinary catheter with continuous bladder irrigation. After assessing that the catheter is patent and is draining freely, the priority nursing intervention is to:
   a. reassure the client that the catheter is draining appropriately.
   b. document the client's complaints and assessment findings.
   c. give the client antispasmodic medication.
   d. notify the physician.

   Rationale: ___The answer is (c). Bladder spasms can cause the client to feel an urge to void. Options (a) and (b) do not address the client's current need. Option (d) is not appropriate at this time.___

2-19 THE PATIENT RECEIVING A BLOOD TRANSFUSION (DEVELOPMENT OF SIGNS AND SYMPTOMS OF A HEMOLYTIC REACTION)

Mr. TA, 34 years old, was admitted after a motor vehicle accident: pedestrian versus car. He sustained multiple injuries throughout his body. He will receive 2 units of whole blood this morning. He has NS 0.9% infusing at TKO rate through a Y-type blood administration set, and he has a 19-gauge cannula in the RFA. The MD orders to infuse each unit over 3 hours. As you get out of the report, the lab notifies you that the first unit of blood is ready.

Prioritize the five **nursing interventions** as you would do them to take care of Mr. TA. Write a number in the box to identify the order of your interventions (#1 = first intervention, #2 = second intervention, etc.) and state a **rationale** for each intervention.

INTERVENTIONS	PRIORITY #	RATIONALE
• Take an initial set of vital signs, assess pain level, pulse ox	☐	_____ _____ _____
• Pick up the blood from the lab	☐	_____ _____ _____
• Assess the IV site	☐	_____ _____ _____
• Start the transfusion	☐	_____ _____ _____
• Verify MD order, blood compatability, and patient ID with another RN at patient bedside (point of care patient identification)	☐	_____ _____ _____

KEY POINTS TO CONSIDER _____

_____

_____

_____

You assess the following during the start of the transfusion on Mr. TA:
1. VS: T 97.6° F, P 80, R 18, BP 136/78 (pretransfusion)
2. VS: T 98.2° F, P 90, R 22, BP 130/70 (15 minutes after the start of the transfusion)
3. No complaints of itching
4. Transfusion rate increased to 100 mL/hr

Integrated Learning Activity: With a partner, **do the following: (1) select** the **one nursing diagnosis** that is a priority at this time, **(2) provide a rationale** for your selection, and **(3) list the nursing interventions** that assist you to meet the needs of the patient.

All of the following nursing diagnoses may apply to Mr. TA:

Risk for infection, Fatigue, Risk for impaired skin integrity, Deficient fluid volume, Deficient knowledge, Anxiety, Risk for injury, Acute pain

Nursing Diagnosis	Rationale	Nursing Interventions

After 20 minutes, Mr. TA's **assessment** includes: Skin flushed, P 120, R 32, BP 100/60, complains of chest pain and chills

Based on the above **assessment,** identify and write the **priority problem** in the box below. Then, starting with the small box labeled **#1, prioritize** the **nursing interventions** for this situation and **identify** your follow-up action plan for Mr. TA.

NURSING INTERVENTIONS

A. Stop the transfusion

B. Inform MD/Lab

C. Save the next voided specimen

D. Start 0.9% NS at TKO rate with new IV tubing

E. Take VS, pulse ox

F. Save the transfusion unit

DECISION-MAKING DIAGRAM

New Action Plan

#1 #2 #3 #4 #5 #6

Priority Problem

NOTES _____

_____

2-20 THE PATIENT WITH NEUTROPENIA (DEVELOPMENT OF SIGNS AND SYMPTOMS OF ACTIVE BLEEDING)

Mrs. K, 50 years old, was admitted 2 days ago with neutropenia. Her current white blood cell count is $750/mm^3$. You note the following from the nursing care Kardex:

VS q4h I & O (✔) Neutropenic precautions (✔) Bone marrow biopsy—today CBC with diff—today Chest x-ray done	Diet: ↑ protein, ↑ calorie (no raw vegetables/fresh fruit) IV: D5W @ 125 mL/hr IV site: RFA (inserted 2 days ago)	Routine medication: Colace 100 mg po daily 0900 PRN medication: Acetaminophen 325 tabs ii q4h po prn for temp greater than 100.4° F

Prioritize the five **nursing interventions** as you would do them to take care of Mrs. K. Write a number in the box to identify the order of your interventions (#1 = first intervention, #2 = second intervention, etc.) and state a **rationale** for each intervention.

INTERVENTIONS	PRIORITY #	RATIONALE
• Wash hands	☐	_____ _____ _____
• Assess the IV site	☐	_____ _____ _____
• Provide fresh water at bedside	☐	_____ _____ _____
• Assess oral mucosa	☐	_____ _____ _____
• Take the vital signs, assess pain level, pulse ox	☐	_____ _____ _____

KEY POINTS TO CONSIDER _____
_____
_____

TWO

Mrs. K is diagnosed with acute leukemia. Your follow-up assessment includes:
1. Hgb 9.8 g/dL, hematocrit 29%
2. White blood cell count 900/mm^3 with an absolute neutrophil count (ANC) 600 cells/μL.
3. Monitoring temperature, oral mucosa
4. Platelet count 100,000/mm^3

Integrated Learning Activity: With a partner, **do the following: (1) select** the **one nursing diagnosis** that is a priority at this time, **(2) provide a rationale** for your selection, and **(3) list the nursing interventions** that assist you to meet the needs of the patient.

All of the following nursing diagnoses may apply to Mrs. K:

Risk for infection, Fatigue, Imbalanced nutrition: less than body requirements, Deficient knowledge, Anxiety, Risk for injury, Impaired oral mucous membrane, Activity intolerance, Risk for impaired skin integrity, Social isolation, Fear, Hopelessness, Impaired physical mobility

Nursing Diagnosis	Rationale	Nursing Interventions

The following day, Mrs. K's **assessment findings** are significant for: Platelet count 30,000/mm^3; bleeding time prolonged, oral petechiae, hemoptysis, tachypnea, dyspnea, and a current nosebleed.

On the basis of the most current **assessment,** identify and write the **priority problem** in the box below. Then, starting with the small box labeled **#1,** prioritize the **nursing interventions** for this situation and **identify** your follow-up action plan for Mrs. K.

NURSING INTERVENTIONS

A. Take the vital signs

B. Assess other site for signs and symptoms of bleeding

C. Assess neurologic status

D. Place in Fowler position

E. Apply direct pressure to nose

F. Inform physician

DECISION-MAKING DIAGRAM

New Action Plan

#1 #2 #3 #4 #5 #6

☐ ☐ ☐ ☐ ☐ ☐

Priority Problem

NOTES _____

_____

2-21 THE PATIENT WITH A HIP FRACTURE (DEVELOPMENT OF SIGNS AND SYMPTOMS OF RESPIRATORY DISTRESS)

Mrs. T, 72 years old, fell at home and was admitted to the hospital with a fracture of the right hip. She was alert and oriented on admission. After the initial workup, she was taken to surgery for an open reduction with internal fixation (ORIF) of her right hip. This is her first postop day. Her right hip dressing has a small amount of dried dark red drainage. She has an IV of $D_5/0.45$ NS at 75 mL/hr, oxygen at 2 L/min/nasal cannula, and is on a clear liquid diet. The neurovascular checks to the right leg are q4h for the first 24 hours. The right leg is warm, pedal pulse present, capillary refill around 2 seconds. IV PCA with morphine sulfate delivering 1 mg/hr continuous infusion. The following medications are ordered: $FeSO_4$ 325 mg po tid with meals (start when on regular diet), docusate sodium 100 mg po daily. The urinary catheter is draining clear urine. Current vital signs are P 80, R 18, BP 110/84. She is very restless and confused this morning.

Prioritize the five interventions according to Mrs. T's current needs. Write a number in the box to identify the order of your interventions (#1 = first intervention, #2 = second intervention, etc.) and state a **rationale** for each intervention.

INTERVENTIONS	PRIORITY #	RATIONALE
• Assess surgical dressing	☐	_____
• Take VS, assess pain level, check pulse ox	☐	_____
• Assess neuro status	☐	_____
• Assess right leg position and body alignment	☐	_____
• Check neurovascular status of right leg (CMST)	☐	_____

KEY POINTS TO CONSIDER _____

_____

During the follow-up assessment for the **first postop day,** you note the following:
1. Pedal pulse present; weak in the right foot, stronger on left foot
2. Hemoglobin 10.5 g/dL and hematocrit 32%
3. Bowel sounds hypoactive in all quadrants
4. Crackles in the lower bases of the lung

Integrated Learning Activity: With a partner, **do the following: (1) select** the **one nursing diagnosis** that is a priority at this time, **(2) provide a rationale** for your selection, and **(3) list the nursing interventions** that assist you to meet the needs of the patient.

All of the following nursing diagnoses may apply to Mrs. T:

Acute pain, Risk for infection, Risk for impaired skin integrity, Impaired urinary elimination, Impaired gas exchange, Fatigue, Impaired physical mobility, Ineffective peripheral tissue perfusion, Acute confusion, Constipation

Nursing Diagnosis	Rationale	Nursing Interventions

On the second postop day Mrs. T is still very confused and is trying to get out of bed. She has bilateral scattered crackles in the lungs, labored breathing, shortness of breath on exertion, R 32, P 108, pulse ox 92%, and a productive cough, whitish sputum. Skin cool, pallor.

Based on the most current situation, identify and write the **priority problem** in the box below. Then, starting with the small box labeled **#1, prioritize** the **nursing interventions** for this situation and **identify** your plan for follow-up care for Mrs. T.

NURSING INTERVENTIONS   **DECISION-MAKING DIAGRAM**

A. Monitor P, R, BP q5min

B. Check oxygen saturation continuously

C. Stay with patient

D. Administer O_2 per nasal cannula

E. Call physician

F. Prepare to transfer patient

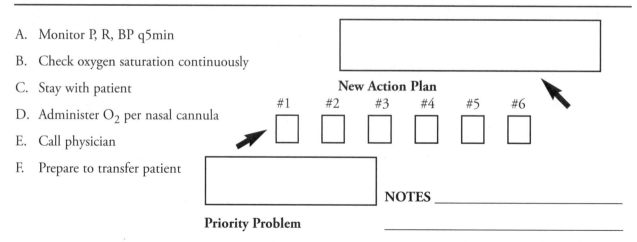

New Action Plan

#1 #2 #3 #4 #5 #6

Priority Problem

NOTES _____

_____

APPLYING CRITICAL THINKING SKILLS TO TEST QUESTIONS

INSTRUCTIONS: Circle the one best answer for each test question. Write your rationale for selecting the answer. To enhance your learning and test-taking skills, discuss your answer and rationale with a partner. The answer and the rationale can be found on the back of this page.

1. The nurse is caring for an 82-year-old client who is 1 day postop left hip replacement. The client has a primary IV infusing at 100 mL/hr, a patient-controlled analgesic device, and a urinary catheter. After assessing the client, the nurse determines that the client is pleasant and cooperative but forgetful. In the afternoon, the nurse notes that the client has become increasingly restless. It is most important of the nurse to:
   a. apply a vest restraint.
   b. notify the physician.
   c. check the patient-controlled analgesic device.
   d. assess the client's medical history for dementia.

   Rationale: _____
   _____
   _____
   _____
   _____

2. The nurse is delegating the care of a 79-year-old client 2 days postop hip replacement to a nursing assistant who routinely works on a medical unit. Which instruction given to the nursing assistant is of priority initially?
   a. Have the client cough and deep breathe q2h.
   b. Total the intake and output at 1400.
   c. Use a fracture bedpan for the client.
   d. Wash the client's skin with a mild soap.

   Rationale: _____
   _____
   _____
   _____
   _____

3. The nurse is assisting a client to get out of a chair after having a right hip replacement 3 days ago. The client suddenly complains of pain and tells the nurse that it hurts too much to walk. Which nursing intervention is of priority?
   a. Encourage the client to put most of the weight on the left leg.
   b. Support the client's right side as the client is asked to stand up.
   c. Assess the client's right hip and leg.
   d. Administer pain medication.

   Rationale: _____
   _____
   _____
   _____
   _____

ANSWER KEY FOR
APPLYING CRITICAL THINKING SKILLS TO TEST QUESTIONS

HELPFUL HINTS: Read all test questions carefully. Identify key words in the question that will guide you in answering the question. In these test questions the **key words** to consider are **"most important," "priority initially,"** and **"priority."** Compare your rationale with the one in the test question.

1. The nurse is caring for an 82-year-old client who is 1 day postop left hip replacement. The client has a primary IV infusing at 100 mL/hr, a patient-controlled analgesic device, and a urinary catheter. After assessing the client, the nurse determines that the client is pleasant and cooperative but forgetful. In the afternoon, the nurse notes that the client has become increasingly restless. It is most important of the nurse to:
   a. apply a vest restraint.
   b. notify the physician.
   c. check the patient-controlled analgesic device.
   d. assess the client's medical history for dementia.

   Rationale: The answer is (c). Pain may be a contributing factor to the client's restlessness. The patient-controlled analgesic device should be checked to see whether the client has used it to control the pain. Options (a), (b), and (d) are not appropriate interventions.

2. The nurse is delegating the care of a 79-year-old client 2 days postop hip replacement to a nursing assistant who routinely works on a medical unit. Which instruction given to the nursing assistant is of priority initially?
   a. Have the client cough and deep breathe q2h.
   b. Total the intake and output at 1400.
   c. Use a fracture bedpan for the client.
   d. Wash the client's skin with a mild soap.

   Rationale: The answer is (c). A fractured bedpan will minimize putting stress on the hip area and prevent hip dislocation. Options (a), (b), and (d) are important, but instructing a new nursing assistant on how to prevent complications on an unfamiliar unit is of priority.

3. The nurse is assisting a client to get out of a chair after having a right hip replacement 3 days ago. The client suddenly complains of pain and tells the nurse that it hurts too much to walk. Which nursing intervention is of priority?
   a. Encourage the client to put most of the weight on the left leg.
   b. Support the client's right side as the client is asked to stand up.
   c. Assess the client's right hip and leg.
   d. Administer pain medication.

   Rationale: The answer is (c). Increased pain may indicate hip dislocation. Options (a), (b), and (d) are good interventions, but the nurse should assess the surgical site before continuing with any other intervention.

2-22 THE PATIENT WITH A FRACTURED TIBIA (DEVELOPMENT OF SIGNS AND SYMPTOMS OF COMPARTMENT SYNDROME)

Mr. W, 26 years old, was admitted with a left fractured tibia. He was taken to surgery and is now being transferred to the orthopedic unit. He has a long leg cast on the left leg. His postop orders are transcribed to the nursing care Kardex:

VS q4h I & O (✓) Neurovascular cks (circ. movement, sensation, temp) q2h for 48 hours Elevate left leg on (1) pillow	1 L D5W q10h—discontinue when taking fluids well Teach crutch walking in AM by physical therapy	Diet: Clear liquids → Reg. Medications IV pump PCA: Hydromorphone 0.2 mg/hr continuous infusion

You are assigned to Mr. W as he is taken into his room. You note that he is alert, the left leg cast is damp and clean, and the IV and PCA are infusing into his right hand.

Prioritize the five **nursing interventions** as you would do them to take care of Mr. W. Write a number in the box to identify the order of your interventions (#1 = first intervention, #2 = second intervention, etc.) and state a **rationale** for each intervention.

INTERVENTIONS	PRIORITY #	RATIONALE
• Take VS, assess pain level, pulse ox	☐	_____
• Neurovascular assessment of both extremities	☐	_____
• Assess cast for dryness, signs of drainage, and sharp edges	☐	_____
• Use palms of hands to elevate cast on a pillow	☐	_____
• Teach isometric exercises	☐	_____

KEY POINTS TO CONSIDER _____

On the morning of the first postop day, you note the following:
1. Mr. W states his pain level is 3 out of 10
2. Left pedal pulses present, edema 2+
3. Capillary refill greater than 2 seconds, moves left toes
4. Taking fluids and voiding quantity sufficient
5. MD orders CPK, LDH, and AST

Integrated Learning Activity: With a partner, **do the following: (1) select** the **one nursing diagnosis** that is a priority at this time, **(2) provide a rationale** for your selection, and **(3) list the nursing interventions** that assist you to meet the needs of the patient.

All of the following nursing diagnoses may apply to Mr. W:

> Risk for injury, Deficient knowledge, Risk for infection, Risk for impaired skin integrity, Impaired physical mobility, Fear, Ineffective peripheral tissue perfusion, Acute pain, Activity intolerance, Impaired tissue integrity, Anxiety, Risk for peripheral neurovascular dysfunction

Nursing Diagnosis	Rationale	Nursing Interventions

Mr. W refuses lunch and you assess: complaints of increased pain 8 out of 10, especially with elevation of the leg, numbness and tingling, left pedal pulse weak, cool

On the basis of this new information, identify and write the **priority problem** in the box below. Then, starting with the small box labeled **#1**, prioritize the **nursing interventions** for this situation and **identify** your follow-up action plan for Mr. W.

NURSING INTERVENTIONS

A. Inform MD stat

B. Prepare to have cast bivalved

C. Ensure that left extremity is at heart level

D. Monitor left pedal pulse

E. Take VS

F. Stay with patient

DECISION-MAKING DIAGRAM

New Action Plan

#1   #2   #3   #4   #5   #6

☐   ☐   ☐   ☐   ☐   ☐

Priority Problem

NOTES _____

_____

2-23 THE PATIENT WITH CATARACT SURGERY (DEVELOPMENT OF SIGNS AND SYMPTOMS OF INTRAOCULAR PRESSURE)

Mrs. G, 72 years old, has senile cataracts and has been instilling mydriatic eye drops. Her vision has progressively worsened and she is scheduled today for a right cataract extraction in the outpatient clinic. The MD orders the following preop preparation: NPO; instill mydriatic and cycloplegic eye drops 1 hour before surgery; diazepam 5 mg po 1 hour before surgery. Mrs. G arrives at the outpatient clinic at 0800 and she is scheduled for surgery at 1000.

Prioritize the five **nursing interventions** as you would do them to take care of Mrs. G. Write a number in the box to identify the order of your interventions (#1 = first intervention, #2 = second intervention, etc.) and state a **rationale** for each intervention.

INTERVENTIONS	PRIORITY #	RATIONALE
• Provide information regarding preop preparation	☐	_____
• Begin to instill ordered eye drops	☐	_____
• Have patient void	☐	_____
• Take VS	☐	_____
• Ensure that the surgical consent is signed before initiating preop preparation	☐	_____

KEY POINTS TO CONSIDER _____

_____

Mrs. G had an intraocular lens implant and is taken to the recovery room. She has an eye patch on her right eye and you assess the following:

1. No complaints of pain, P 88, BP 130/82
2. Eye patch clean and dry
3. Readily responds to verbal stimuli

Integrated Learning Activity: With a partner, **do the following: (1) select** the **one nursing diagnosis** that is a priority at this time, **(2) provide a rationale** for your selection, and **(3) list the nursing interventions** that assist you to meet the needs of the patient.

All of the following nursing diagnoses may apply to Mrs. G:

> Risk for injury, Deficient knowledge, Fear, Anxiety, Risk for infection, Ineffective health maintenance, Impaired home maintenance

Nursing Diagnosis	Rationale	Nursing Interventions

One hour **postop** you assess Mrs. G and note the following: complaints of right brow pain, anxious, P 110, BP 128/80, coughing, and complaints of nausea

Based on the **postop** assessment, identify and write the **priority problem** in the box below. Then, starting with the small box labeled **#1, prioritize** the **nursing interventions** for this situation and **identify** your follow-up action plan for Mrs. G.

NURSING INTERVENTIONS

A. Avoid rapid head movement

B. Administered antiemetic if ordered

C. Document findings/nursing care

D. Notify MD

E. Recheck pulse and BP

F. Stay with Mrs. G

DECISION-MAKING DIAGRAM

New Action Plan

#1   #2   #3   #4   #5   #6

Priority Problem

NOTES _____

_____

2-24 THE PATIENT WITH A SEIZURE DISORDER (DEVELOPMENT OF SEIZURE ACTIVITY)

Mr. M, 20 years old, fell at home and was brought to the emergency department after it was noticed that he had lost consciousness for a few seconds. In the emergency department he indicated that he did not remember falling. His family history is significant for seizure disorders. Diagnostic studies were ordered and included an electroencephalogram, magnetic resonance imaging, serum blood glucose, complete blood cell count, blood urea nitrogen, and urinalysis drug screening. He was just transferred to the neurology unit from the emergency department. The current MD orders include seizure precautions, bed rest, soft diet, saline lock, VS, and neurologic checks q4h.

Prioritize the following **nursing interventions** as you would do them to initially take care of Mr. M. Write a number in the box to identify the order of your interventions (#1 = first intervention, #2 = second intervention, etc.) and state a **rationale** for each intervention.

INTERVENTIONS	PRIORITY #	RATIONALE
• Orient Mr. M to his room	☐	_____
• Assess neurologic status	☐	_____
• Implement seizure precautions	☐	_____
• Obtain admitting history	☐	_____
• Inform of pertinent MD orders	☐	_____

KEY POINTS TO CONSIDER _____

_____

_____

Mr. M is diagnosed with a seizure disorder and is started on divalproex sodium. In speaking with Mr. M you gather the following:

1. Mr. M says that he has had similar episodes but never told anyone.
2. He remembers seeing "spots" before the episode.
3. No one in his family talked much about the relative who had seizures.

Integrated Learning Activity: With a partner, **do the following: (1) select** the **one nursing diagnosis** that is a priority at this time, **(2) provide a rationale** for your selection, and **(3) list the nursing interventions** that assist you to meet the needs of the patient.

All of the following nursing diagnoses may apply to Mr. M:

Ineffective coping, Ineffective airway clearance, Risk for injury, Readiness for enhanced knowledge: seizure disorder, Social isolation, Fear, Anxiety, Ineffective health maintenance, Risk for aspiration

Nursing Diagnosis	Rationale	Nursing Interventions

Several hours after admission, you hear a "cry" coming from Mr. M's room. You assess the following as you walk into the room: Tonic-clonic movements of the body, loss of consciousness, excessive salivation, some cyanosis, urinary incontinence, teeth clenched with cessation of tonic-clonic movements after 3 minutes.

On the basis of the situation just described, identify and write the **priority problem** in the box below. Then, starting with the small box labeled **#1**, prioritize the **nursing interventions** for this situation and identify your follow-up action plan for Mr. M.

NURSING INTERVENTIONS

DECISION-MAKING DIAGRAM

A. Maintain a quiet environment

B. Assess for injury

C. Check airway patency

D. Document findings

E. Turn to side

F. Reorient patient

New Action Plan

#1 #2 #3 #4 #5 #6

Priority Problem

NOTES _____

_____

APPLYING CRITICAL THINKING SKILLS TO TEST QUESTIONS

INSTRUCTIONS: Circle the one best answer for each test question. Write your rationale for selecting the answer. To enhance your learning and test-taking skills, discuss your answer and rationale with a partner. The answer and the rationale can be found on the back of this page.

1. The nurse documents the following after observing a client have a tonic-clonic seizure: "0930 Found client having jerky, involuntary movements of upper and lower extremities lasting 2 minutes, frothy saliva oozing from mouth, incontinent of urine." Which statement best describes the nurse's documentation? The documentation:
   a. is appropriate and describes the observations seen.
   b. should include the client's response and nursing interventions.
   c. should just indicate that the client had a tonic-clonic seizure.
   d. is lacking whether the client had an aura experience before the seizure.

   Rationale: _____
   _____
   _____
   _____
   _____

2. The nurse admits a client who is having uncontrolled generalized tonic-clonic seizures. In planning for potential complications, which nursing intervention is of priority?
   a. Have a tongue blade next to the client's bed.
   b. Have suction equipment available.
   c. Maintain side rails up at all times.
   d. Maintain a quiet environment.

   Rationale: _____
   _____
   _____
   _____
   _____

3. The nurse is caring for a client who is on phenytoin (Dilantin) 200 mg po tid and phenobarbital 20 mg po tid. Which assessment finding is most indicative of a common side effect of these medications?
   a. Gums red and swollen
   b. Complaints of constipation
   c. Respiratory depression
   d. Skin rash

   Rationale: _____
   _____
   _____
   _____
   _____

HELPFUL HINTS: Read all test questions carefully. Identify key words in the question that will guide you in answering the question. In these test questions the **key words** to consider are **"best," "priority,"** and **"most indicative."** Compare your rationale with the one in the test question.

1. The nurse documents the following after observing a client have a tonic-clonic seizure: "0930 Found client having jerky, involuntary movements of upper and lower extremities lasting 2 minutes, frothy saliva oozing from mouth, incontinent of urine." Which statement best describes the nurse's documentation? The documentation:
   a. is appropriate and describes the observations seen.
   b. should include the client's response and nursing interventions.
   c. should just indicate that the client had a tonic-clonic seizure.
   d. is lacking whether the client had an aura experience before the seizure.

   Rationale: The answer is (b). Documentation should include what is observed, the nursing interventions, and the client's response/reaction. Options (a), (c), and (d) do not include all the components necessary for legal documentation.

2. The nurse admits a client who is having uncontrolled generalized tonic-clonic seizures. In planning for potential complications, which nursing intervention is of priority?
   a. Have a tongue blade next to the client's bed.
   b. Have suction equipment available.
   c. Maintain side rails up at all times.
   d. Maintain a quiet environment.

   Rationale: The answer is (b). Suction equipment is necessary to clear oral secretions after the seizure and prevent aspiration. Options (c) and (d) are important, but preventing aspiration is of priority. Option (a) is not a current intervention.

3. The nurse is caring for a client who is on phenytoin (Dilantin) 200 mg po tid and phenobarbital 20 mg po tid. Which assessment finding is most indicative of a common side effect of these medications?
   a. Gums red and swollen
   b. Complaints of constipation
   c. Respiratory depression
   d. Skin rash

   Rationale: The answer is (a). Gingival hyperplasia is a common side effect seen with the administration of phenytoin. Meticulous oral hygiene is an important intervention. Option (b) is not a common side effect. Option (c) is a toxic reaction to phenobarbital, and option (d) is a toxic reaction to phenytoin.

2-25 THE PATIENT WITH A DO-NOT-RESUSCITATE ORDER (DEVELOPMENT OF SIGNS AND SYMPTOMS OF IMPENDING DEATH)

Mr. B, 83 years old, has terminal esophageal cancer. The following pertinent information is found in the nursing care rand:

Activity: Bed rest Vital signs: q4h Oral suction prn Lives with son Hospital Day: #4	PEG tube insertion: 3 days ago Formula full strength: 50 mL/hr Ck residual q4h, if greater than 100 mL, hold feeding for 1 hour PRN medications: Morphine sulfate 2 mg direct IV injection q2h prn pain	IV: 0.9% NS q12h Urinary catheter inserted on admission I & O q8h Code status: DNR

The 7:00 AM handoff report indicates that his current respirations are 10 and he last received morphine sulfate at 6:00 AM. Residual at that time was 125 mL; tube feeding was stopped. IV has 200 mL left.

Prioritize the five **nursing interventions** as you would do them to initially take care of Mr. B. Write a number in the box to identify the order of your interventions (#1= first intervention, #2 = second intervention, etc.) and state a **rationale** for each intervention.

INTERVENTIONS	PRIORITY #	RATIONALE
• Assess PEG tube residual	☐	_____
• Take VS and pain level	☐	_____
• Assess IV site and IV fluid level	☐	_____
• Perform a body system assessment	☐	_____
• Assess patency of urinary catheter and output	☐	_____

KEY POINTS TO CONSIDER _____

At 11:00 AM Mr. B manifested the following signs and symptoms:

1. VS: P 76, R14, BP 118/64, pulse ox 93%, pain level difficult to assess
2. Responds appropriately but is weak and lethargic, no grimacing
3. Urine is dark yellow; output 125 mL since 7:00 AM
4. Shortness of breath when turning; irregular breathing pattern

Integrated Learning Activity: With a partner, **do the following: (1) select** the **one nursing diagnosis** that is a priority at this time, **(2) provide a rationale** for your selection, and **(3) list the nursing interventions** that assist you to meet the needs of the patient.

All of the following nursing diagnoses may apply to Mr. B:

Risk for infection, Acute pain, Anxiety, Impaired gas exchange, Imbalanced nutrition: less than body requirements, Risk for deficient fluid volume, Risk for impaired skin integrity, Ineffective peripheral tissue perfusion, Activity intolerance, Powerlessness, Social isolation

Nursing Diagnosis	Rationale	Nursing Interventions

At **2:00 PM** Mr. B is unresponsive to verbal stimuli. You assessed: VS: P 36, R 9, BP 80/50, pulse ox 86%. Urine output unchanged since 11:00 AM. Lower extremities cool with cyanosis.

Based on the **2:00 PM** assessment, identify and write the **priority problem** in the box below. Then, starting with the small box labeled **#1**, prioritize the **nursing interventions** for this situation and **identify** your plan for follow-up care for Mr. B.

NURSING INTERVENTIONS

A. Monitor VS

B. Check NCP for religious/cultural requests

C. Report findings to physician

D. Notify relatives

E. Provide comfort measures

F. Document findings

DECISION-MAKING DIAGRAM

New Action Plan

#1 #2 #3 #4 #5 #6

Priority Problem

NOTES _____

_____

2-26 LEGAL CONSIDERATIONS
(MEDICATION ERROR)

Mrs. L is 1 day postop total abdominal hysterectomy. She is 42 years old. Morphine sulfate 5 mg is ordered direct IV injection q3h prn pain. She is on a clear liquid diet and has not voided since the urinary catheter was removed at noon. She is ambulating with assistance to the bathroom. The abdominal dressing is stained with dried dark red drainage. VS at noon are T 99° F, P 82, R 22, BP 130/76, pulse ox 96%. Fine crackles are audible in the lower bases of the lung fields. It is 4:00 PM and she is requesting pain medication. She states her pain level is 4 out of 10. Her last pain shot was administered at 2:00 PM. An incentive spirometer is at the bedside.

Prioritize the following **nursing interventions** as you, the nurse, would do them to initially take care of Mrs. L. Write a number in the box to identify the order of your interventions (#1 = first intervention, #2 = second intervention, etc.) and state a **rationale** for each intervention.

INTERVENTIONS	PRIORITY #	RATIONALE
• Inform Mrs. L that the pain medication is not due for another hour	☐	_____ _____ _____
• Cough and deep breathe; demonstrate abdominal splinting; use incentive spirometer q1h	☐	_____ _____ _____
• Ambulate to the bathroom	☐	_____ _____ _____
• Take VS	☐	_____ _____ _____
• Assess abdomen and surgical dressing	☐	_____ _____ _____

KEY POINTS TO CONSIDER _____
_____
_____
_____

Mrs. L voids 400 mL after ambulating to the bathroom and states that she feels much better. She relates the following to you:

1. Her mother had a hysterectomy but died 10 days after from surgical complications.
2. She is glad that she does not have to worry about irregular periods any more.
3. She fully trusts her doctor but wonders whether the right thing was done.
4. She lives alone.

Integrated Learning Activity: With a partner, **do the following: (1) select** the **one nursing diagnosis** that is a priority at this time, **(2) provide a rationale** for your selection, and **(3) list the nursing interventions** that assist you to meet the needs of the patient.

All of the following nursing diagnoses may apply to Mrs. L:

> Risk for infection, Acute pain, Anxiety, Ineffective breathing pattern, Imbalanced nutrition: less than body requirements, Disturbed body image, Sexual dysfunction, Impaired skin integrity, Risk for activity intolerance, Deficient knowledge

Nursing Diagnosis	Rationale	Nursing Interventions

At 6:00 PM Mrs. L states that she is having pain. Mrs. L's pain is at a level of 8 out of 10. She has not received any pain medication since 2:00 PM. You take out an ampule labeled hydromorphone 10 mg/mL and administer 0.5 mL to Mrs. L. After the administration of the hydromorphone you realize that hydromorphone is not morphine sulfate.

Based on the situation just described, identify and write the **priority problem** in the box below. Then, starting with the small box labeled **#1, prioritize** the **nursing interventions** for this situation and **identify** your follow-up action plan for Mrs. L.

NURSING INTERVENTIONS   DECISION-MAKING DIAGRAM

A. Stay with the patient

B. Document drug and amount given

C. Monitor respiratory depression and circulatory collapse

D. Fill out an incident report

E. Notify your RN and instructor stat

F. Notify physician stat

New Action Plan

#1   #2   #3   #4   #5   #6

Priority Problem

NOTES _____

3-1 SMALL BOWEL RESECTION WITH POSTOP CARE

Handoff report at 0700:

"Mr. A, a 72-year-old male, is 2 days postop small bowel resection. His NG tube is connected to continuous low wall suction and is draining dark brown fluid. Vital signs at 0600: T 99.6° F, P 90, R 28, BP 160/94, pulse ox 94%. IV D5/0.45 NS with 20 mEq KCl infusing at 125 mL into the right forearm. He is using the PCA with relief. He slept most of the night and is now sitting in a chair. SOB was noted when he was transferred to the chair. There are 300 mL left in the IV."

Mr. A's current **flowcharts** contain the following information:

Medication Record	
Routine	**Time Due**
Digoxin 0.25 mg IVP daily	0900
Furosemide 20 mg IVP daily	0900
Timolol 0.25% gtt **i** both eyes BID	1000
Pantoprazole 40 mg IVPB daily	1000
Gentamicin 80 mg IVPB q8h	1400
PRN	
PCA (morphine sulfate 0.7 mg on demand; lock out 8 min, dose limit 20 mg in 4 hours)	

Intake and Output Record

Night Shift @ 0600

Intake			Output		
PO	=	0	UA Void	=	0
			Foley	=	200
IV	=	1000	N/G	=	600
IVPB	=	100			

⚡ **Integrated Learning Activity:** With a partner, **use the clinical situation and the flowcharts** to:

1. Identify the pertinent patient information made known to you in the *report*. →	2. Identify the pertinent patient information made known to you in the *flowcharts*. →	3. Review the data in columns 1 and 2 and identify information that needs follow-up.

It is 0730 when the handoff report is completed. **Prioritize** your plan of care for the morning:

Time	Plan of Nursing Care

1200 nursing assessment: Oriented ×3, skin WNL, capillary refill less than 3 sec, turgor good, mucous membranes moist, pinkish, T 99° F, P 88 and slightly irregular, R 20, BP 164/94, pulse ox 96%. NG draining brownish fluid 100 mL since 0800. Bowel sounds present ×4, abd soft. Foley catheter draining clear yellow urine.

Mr. A has minimal complaints and is visited by the physician at 1200. The physician leaves the following orders:

> Remove Foley now
> Enc. incentive spirometer q1h ×10
> Discontinue NG tube
> Discontinue furosemide
> Discontinue IV digoxin, start digoxin 0.25 mg po daily
> Hgb & Hct today
> Clear liquid diet

1. Identify the nursing interventions that require immediate follow-up.	2. Identify the nursing actions that you can delegate/assign to unlicensed personnel.

Critical reflection: To promote **safe nursing practice,** the handoff report at 0700 and the flowcharts:

☐ communicated sufficient information to provide continuous care to the patient.

☐ lacked the following: _____

_____

_____

3-2 PATIENT WITH GI BLEED AND ETOH ABUSE

Handoff report at 7:00 AM:

"The patient is 43 years old and was admitted yesterday from the ED after experiencing GI bleeding. He is NPO and has an NG tube connected to continuous low wall suction. The NG has drained 100 mL of dark reddish drainage. Vital signs at 6:00 AM are T 97.4° F, P 96, R 18, BP 130/86, pulse ox 96%. A unit of whole blood is infusing and should be complete by 9:00 AM. His current Hgb is 8.6. He does have a history of ETOH abuse and has been more restless this morning."

The patient's current **flowcharts** contain the following information:

Patient Care Kardex
IV: D5/0.9 NS c̄ 10 mL MVI @ 100 mL/hr into RFA #20 g
IV site: #18 g LFA for blood administration
Give two units of whole blood today #1 ☑   #2 ☐
H & H in the AM ☐
BRP with assistance only Monitor for seizure activity
Routine Medication: Famotidine 20 mg q12h IVPB 1000-2200

Intake and Output Record

Night Shift @ 0600

Intake			Output		
PO	=	0	UA void	=	525
			NG	=	100
IV	=	600			
0.9% NS	=	50			
Transfusion	=	50			

Integrated Learning Activity: With a partner, **use the clinical situation and the flowcharts** to:

1. Identify the pertinent patient information made known to you in the *report*.	2. Identify the pertinent patient information made known to you in the *flowcharts*.	3. Review the data in columns 1 and 2 and identify information that needs follow-up.

It is 7:30 AM when the handoff report is completed. **Prioritize** your plan of care for the morning:

Time	Plan of Nursing Care

10:00 AM nursing assessment: Anxious, restless, pulled out NG tube. Physician called. VS: P 100, R 26, BP 146/90. Vomited 20 mL bright red fluid. Bowel sounds present ×4, abd soft. Transfusion #2 infusing at 25 gtt/min.

The physician calls back and gives the following telephone orders:

    Oxygen at 2 L/min/NP
    Reinsert NG tube
    ABG, serum electrolytes Mg^{++}, BG, serum ammonia level, BUN
    VS and neuro checks q2h
    Chlordiazepoxide HCl 50 mg IV push stat

1. Identify the nursing interventions that require immediate follow-up.	2. Identify the nursing actions that you can delegate/assign to unlicensed personnel.

Critical reflection: To implement safe nursing interventions, identify the signs and symptoms associated with alcohol withdrawal syndrome:

Stage I: _____

Stage II: _____

Stage III: _____

Stage IV: _____

3-3 PATIENT WITH DEHYDRATION, FEVER, DO-NOT-RESUSCITATE ORDER

Handoff report at 1600:

"The patient was admitted today for dehydration. She is 88 years old and has a stage IV pressure ulcer on her sacrum. A wet-to-dry dressing is clean and intact. A pressure ulcer with eschar is on her left heel. She weighs 90 pounds and she refused her lunch. An IV was started at 1400. You have 750 mL credit. She is a sweet little lady, quiet, and at times forgetful. Her admission lab results just came in, her Hgb is 9.6, Hct 27, WBC 11,000, and K^+ 4.5. I have not called the physician."

The patient's current **flowcharts** contain the following information:

Patient Care Kardex
VS q4h   Diet: Pureed
HOH
Siderails ↑ ×2
W-D Drsg c̄ 0.9 NS q12h   0800 - 2000
IV: D5/0.9 NS at 75 mL/hr
IV site: R hand #24 g cannula
Medication: Colace 100 mg po daily
Do not resuscitate (DNR)

Intake and Output Record		
Day Shift — 8 hour		
Intake		**Output**
PO = 50		UA = inc ×2
IV = 250		

⚡ **Integrated Learning Activity:** With a partner, **use the clinical situation and the flowcharts** to:

1. Identify the pertinent patient information made known to you in the *report*.	2. Identify the pertinent patient information made known to you in the *flowcharts*.	3. Review the data in columns 1 and 2 and identify information that needs follow-up.

It is 1630 when the handoff report is completed. **Prioritize** your plan of care for the next 4 hours:

Time	Plan of Nursing Care

At 2000 the nursing assistant reports that the patient is restless and trying to get out of bed. You document the following assessment: Speech incoherent, skin warm, flushed. VS: T 101° F, P 92, R 24, BP 108/60, pulse ox 88%. Incontinent of dark-colored urine with strong odor. Physician called. The following telephone orders are given:

VS q2h, I & O
Acetaminophen 325 mg po q4h prn temperature greater than 100.4° F
Enc. fluid intake
Ceftriaxone 1 g IVPB qAM

1. Identify the nursing interventions that require immediate follow-up.	2. Identify the nursing actions that you can delegate/assign to unlicensed personnel.

Critical reflection: To promote patient-centered care, list nursing interventions that you could independently implement for this patient:

_____

_____

_____

_____

_____

_____

_____

_____

_____

3-4 PATIENT WITH FRACTURED TIBIA AND ASTHMA

Handoff report at 2300:

"The patient in Room 205 was admitted with a fractured right tibia and is 1 day postop. He has a cast on. He has been quiet most of the evening. He just started coughing and is experiencing some SOB. He says he has a history of asthma and that he gets this way every now and then. I did not detect any wheezing. Vital signs are T 98.8° F, P 90, R 28, BP 140/88, pulse ox 92%, pain level 3 out of 10 on the pain scale. Circulation, movement, and sensation are WNL in the right leg."

The patient's current **flowcharts** contain the following information:

Nursing Care Rand

Up in chair   Diet: Regular

PT to teach crutch walking ☑

IV: Saline lock #20g RFA

Circ. movement, sensation and temp. (CMST) right leg q4h
Elevate leg on one pillow

PRN Medication:
PCA - morphine sulfate 1 mg on demand;
8 min lock out; 4 hour dose limit = 30 mg

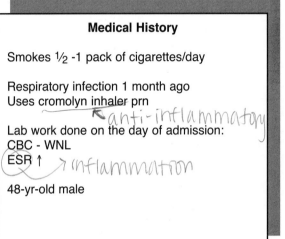

Medical History

Smokes ½ -1 pack of cigarettes/day

Respiratory infection 1 month ago
Uses cromolyn inhaler prn   *← anti-inflammatory*

Lab work done on the day of admission:
CBC - WNL
ESR ↑   *→ inflammation*

48-yr-old male

Integrated Learning Activity: With a partner, **use the clinical situation and the flowcharts** to:

1. Identify the pertinent patient information made known to you in the *report*.	2. Identify the pertinent patient information made known to you in the *flowcharts*.	3. Review the data in columns 1 and 2 and identify information that needs follow-up.
- hx of asthma - SOB / coughing - R: 28 - BP: 140/88 - O₂: 92%	- smokes ½ -1 pk/day - resp. infection 1mth. ago - uses cromolyn inhaler prn. - PCA pump - ↑ ESR	

It is 2330 as you leave the report room. **Prioritize** your plan of care for the next 3 hours:

Time	Plan of Nursing Care

0200 nursing assessment: The patient is beginning to cough more frequently and complains of chest tightness. Respiratory assessment indicates inspiratory and expiratory wheezes in bilateral lungs. You call the physician and obtain the following telephone orders:

IV D5/0.9 NS at 125 mL/hr 5
Oxygen at 2 L/min/NP 1
Albuterol inhaler 2 puffs q4h (rescue inhaler) 2
Metaproterenol nebulizer treatment 0.3 mL (5%) in 2.5 mL NS q4h prn 3
ABG, sputum for eosinophils 7
Methylprednisolone sodium 125 mg IVP q6h 6
Check oxygen saturation with pulse oximeter q2h 4
Call physician with ABG results 8

What would you do first?

1. Identify the nursing interventions that require immediate follow-up.	2. Identify the nursing actions that you can delegate/assign to unlicensed personnel.

Critical reflection: To promote patient-centered care, list nursing interventions that you could independently implement for this patient:

3-5 PATIENT WITH PANCREATITIS AND CENTRAL LINE

Handoff report at 3:00 PM:

"Mrs. C, 42 years old, was admitted earlier today with the diagnosis of acute pancreatitis. She had midepigastric pain with nausea and vomiting on admission. Her latest vital signs are T 38° C, P 108, R 26, BP 110/60, pulse ox 97%. Bowel sounds are hypoactive. I gave her 5 mg of morphine sulfate at 2:00 PM. A central line was inserted; you have 800 mL left in the IV of lactated Ringer's. The NG is draining brownish fluid."

Mrs. C's current **flowcharts** contain the following information:

Patient Care Kardex	
VS: q4h	Diet: NPO
O_2 @ 3 L/min/NP	
Pulse oximetry q4h	
IV: Lactated Ringer's @150 mL/hr	
Right subclavian central line double lumen	
NG tube to low cont suction ☑	
ABG in AM ☐	
BG, CBC, K^+, Na^+, Cl^-, CO_2, Mg^{++}, Ca^{++} in AM ☐	
Abd CT scan @ 6 PM today	
Routine Medication:	
Famotidine 20 mg q12h IVPB 1000 - 2200	
PRN Medication:	
Morphine sulfate 5 mg direct IV injection q3h prn pain	

Admission Lab Data	
Se Amylase	350 units/L
Se Lipase	260 units/L
Hgb	11.6 g/dL
Hct	32%
WBC	18,000/mm³
LDH	300 units/L
AST	80 units/L
BG	200 mg/dL

Integrated Learning Activity: With a partner, **use the clinical situation and the flowcharts** to:

1. Identify the pertinent patient information made known to you in the *report*.	2. Identify the pertinent patient information made known to you in the *flowcharts*.	3. Review the data in columns 1 and 2 and identify information that needs follow-up.

It is 4:00 PM; prioritize your plan of care for the next 3 hours:

Time	Plan of Nursing Care

At 8:30 PM the nursing assistant informs you that Mrs. C is complaining of pain and is restless. You note that she has not had a pain shot in the last 3 hours. You walk into the room to assess her and to give her the pain medication injection. She turns over quickly and pulls out the central line.

1. Identify the nursing interventions that you would implement immediately at the bedside.	2. Identify the follow-up nursing actions. Document the incident in the nurse's notes.
Nurse's Notes	

Critical reflection: Mrs. C is very anxious after the central line was pulled and asks you if she needs to have that "central line" inserted again. To provide patient-centered care at this time, list two questions that would support Mrs. C current needs.

1. _____

2. _____

Copyright © 2014, 2010, 2006, 2003, 1999 by Saunders, an imprint of Elsevier Inc. All rights reserved.

3-6 PATIENT WITH A HEAD TRAUMA

Handoff report at 8:00 AM:

"The patient is a young man who was transferred from the ICU yesterday. He was in a motor vehicle accident (MVA) 14 days ago. He had some head trauma and subsequent evacuation of a subdural hematoma. He is unconscious, unresponsive to painful stimuli, and has flaccid extremities. Pupils round, sluggish reaction to light. He has several abrasions on his face and several bruised areas on his shoulders and chest from the accident. Vital signs are T 97.8° F, P 94, R 24, BP 124/80, pulse ox 94%. Mother at bedside; she questions everything you do."

The patient's current **flowcharts** contain the following information:

Nursing Care Rand
Oral suction prn   Diet: NPO
VS & neuro checks q4h
O$_2$ @ 3 L/min/NP
Seizure precautions   Foley ☑
HOB ↑ 30° at all times   I & O
LBM: _____   PEG tube clamped
IV: TPN at 80 mL/hr via right subclavian central line—triple lumen
Fingerstick BG q6h 1200 - 1800 - 2400 - 0600
Routine Medication:
Dexamethasone 4 mg IVP q6h 1000 - 1600 - 2200 - 0400
PRN Medication:
Dulcolax supp i prn no BM

Medical History
18-year-old high school student involved in a MVA in which he was the driver. Passenger in the car died from injuries. Pt. unconscious on arrival to the ER.
Drug use: Family not aware of any use. Blood alcohol level on admission 0.16%.
Family wants to continue all possible treatment. Not willing to discuss code status at this time.

Integrated Learning Activity: With a partner, **use the clinical situation and the flowcharts** to:

1. Identify the pertinent patient information made known to you in the *report*.	2. Identify the pertinent patient information made known to you in the *flowcharts*.	3. Review the data in columns 1 and 2 and identify information that needs follow-up.

It is 8:30 AM when the handoff report is completed. **Prioritize** your plan of care for the next 3 hours:

Time	Plan of Nursing Care

2:00 PM nursing assessment: Pupil round R ● L ● nonreactive to light. R 12 Cheyne-Stokes, P 80, BP 150/80. Skin warm, jerky movements of the upper extremity noted. The physician writes the following orders:

Oxygen at 12 L/min per non-rebreather mask
Check oxygen saturation q1h
Vital signs q1h
CT scan of the head stat
ABGs stat

1. Identify the nursing interventions that require immediate follow-up.	2. Identify the nursing actions that you can delegate/assign to unlicensed personnel.

Critical reflection: To provide patient-centered care, list how you would support the mother at this time?

3-7 SENSITIVE POSTMORTEM CARE

Handoff report at 8:00 AM:

"The patient is 52 years old and has bone cancer. She has been requesting pain medication every 2 hours. I gave her morphine sulfate 2 mg this morning at 6:30 AM. Her respirations have gone down to 10 during the night. She does not want to be turned. A urinary catheter was inserted in the evening shift. She is a DNR. A family member spent the night with her. Latest vital signs at 6:00 AM are T 97° F, P 66, R 12, BP 128/60."

The patient's current **flowcharts** contain the following information:

Patient Care Kardex	
VS q4h, pulse ox	Diet: DAT
Comfort measures	Foley ☑
IV: Saline lock	I & O
LBM: inc. ×1 sml	
PRN Medication:	
Morphine sulfate 2 mg IVP q2h prn	
Morphine sulfate 4 mg IVP q4h prn if not relieved with morphine sulfate 2 mg	
DNR	

Nurse's Notes

Night shift
11:00 PM   Awake, responds when spoken to. c/o generalized pain, refuses to be turned. Morphine sulfate 2 mg IVP given. - *C. Todd RN*
11:30 R 10, moans when touched, taking sips of water. Mouth care given. — *C. Todd RN*
12:00 AM   Moaning. Daughter upset, crying, states is afraid that mother is going to die. Referral to pastoral care given. — *C. Todd RN*
1:00 2 mg morphine given IVP, lethargic, arousable, R 10, P 60, BP 110/58. *C. Todd RN*
4:30 Pain med. given————— *C. Todd RN*
5:00 Resting ————— *C. Todd RN*
6:00 Lethargic but arousable —— *C. Todd RN*

Integrated Learning Activity: With a partner, **use the clinical situation and the flowcharts** to:

1. Identify the pertinent patient information made known to you in the *report*.	2. Identify the pertinent patient information made known to you in the *flowcharts*.	3. Review the data in columns 1 and 2 and identify information that needs follow-up.

THREE

It is 8:30 AM when the handoff report is completed. **Prioritize** your plan of care for the next 3 hours:

Time	Plan of Nursing Care

At 12:30 PM you return from lunch to learn that the nursing assistant was unable to obtain a pulse on the patient. You assess the following: Unresponsive, skin cool, legs pale with mottling. Pulse not palpable, no apical or BP audible. Family with patient. Physician contacted and pronounced patient dead. Family is making arrangements for a mortuary to pick up the patient within the hour.

1. Identify the nursing interventions that require immediate follow-up.	2. Identify the nursing actions that you can delegate/assign to unlicensed personnel.

Critical reflection: To provide patient-centered care, identify nursing interventions that support the family during this time.

_____

_____

_____

_____

_____

_____

_____

_____

_____

3-8 PATIENT FALLING WITH COMPLICATIONS

Handoff report at 7:00 AM:

"Mrs. F, 79 years old, was in a motor vehicle accident (MVA) 2 days ago in which she fractured her arm. Her right arm is in a cast; circulation, movement, and sensation are fine. She is scheduled to go home this morning. She slept fine and was given Vicodin for pain at 4:30 AM with relief. VS are WNL and pain level is 1-2 at 6:00 AM."

At 7:30 AM, as you complete the handoff reports on your assigned patients, the night nurse tells you that Mrs. F got up to go to the bathroom and fell coming back to bed. She has a slight nosebleed and was given an icepack and assisted back to bed. The physician was called and informed of her falling. He said he would be in later to see her before discharge.

Mrs. F's current **flowcharts** contain the following information:

Nursing Care Rand

VS: q shift   Diet: DAT

LBM: 1 day ago

Discharge this AM
Discharge instructions: Office appt. 2 wk
Vicodin tab i po q4h prn pain

PRN Medication:
Vicodin tab i po q4h prn pain
Diphenhydramine 25 mg po at bedtime q6h prn

Nurse's Notes
Night shift
11:00 PM Awake, oriented x3. Skin warm and dry. Pulse 88, slightly irregular, lung sound diminished bilaterally in the lower bases. Enc. to take deep breaths, used incentive spirometer x5. Right arm with cast, CMS-WNL. Requesting sleeping medication. Diphenhydramine 25 mg po given. Siderails up x2.
——————————— *S. Dolle RN*
1:30 AM Sleeping ————— *S. Dolle RN*
4:30 AM Awake, requesting pain medication CMS-WNL. Vicodin tab i given — *S. Dolle RN*
6:00 Resting comfortably.——— *S. Dolle RN*

Integrated Learning Activity: With a partner, **use the clinical situation and the flowcharts** to:

1. Identify the pertinent patient information made known to you in the *report*.	2. Identify the pertinent patient information made known to you in the *flowcharts*.	3. Review the data in columns 1 and 2 and identify information that needs follow-up.

THREE

It is 7:30 AM; prioritize your plan of care for the next hour:

Time	Plan of Nursing Care

At 8:30 AM you note that Mrs. F is lethargic and very slow to respond to verbal stimuli. Skin is cool with slight cyanosis noted on nail beds. P 110 and irregular, R 14 shallow, pulse ox 92%, BP 90/70, which is lower than her usual of 130/88.

1. Identify the nursing interventions that you would plan to implement immediately.	2. Identify the nursing actions that you can delegate/assign to unlicensed personnel.

Critical reflection: To promote safe nursing practice, the patient report at 0730:

☐ communicated sufficient information regarding the patient's fall and follow-up nursing interventions.

☐ lacked the following: _____

_____

_____

_____

_____

_____

_____

_____

3-9 PATIENT WITH HYPERTENSION AND MEDICATION ERROR

Handoff report at 0700:

You are assigned to the following two patients:

"Mrs. A is 67 years old and has diabetes mellitus type 1 and hypertension. She is in for a pressure ulcer on her right heel. She is on bed rest with the right leg elevated and she only has BRP. There is a wet-to-dry dressing change due at 10:00 AM. VS are stable and her latest BP is 170/108, denies pain, pulse ox 97%."

"Mrs. C is 73 years old and was admitted with dehydration 3 days ago. She is eating and voiding well. There is a possibility that she is going home today. I removed her saline lock; there was some redness at the IV site. She is not on any IV meds, so I decided not to restart. She says that she is going home this afternoon, although there is no order. Her morning vital signs are: T 97° F, P 82, R 18, BP 130/90, pulse ox 98%, pain level 0."

Mrs. A's and Mrs. C's **medication records** contain the following information:

Medication Record	
Patient: Mrs. A	Allergies: None

Routine	**Time**
Humulin N 26 units subcut qAM 30 minutes ac breakfast	0730
Tenormin 25 mg po daily (patient requests this time)	1100
Furosemide 20 mg po bid	1100 - 1700
Ceftazidine 0.5 g IVPB q8h	1000 - 1800 - 0200

PRN Medication
MOM 30 mL prn constipation
Temazepam 30 mg po at bedtime may repeat ×1

Medication Record	
Patient: Mrs. C	Allergies: None

Routine	**Time**
Prazosin 1 mg po qAM	0900
Multivitamin tab i po qAM	0900

PRN Medication
MOM 30 mL po prn constipation

Integrated Learning Activity: With a partner, **use the clinical situation and the flowcharts** to:

1. Identify the pertinent patient information made known to you in the *report*.	2. Identify the pertinent patient information made known to you in the *flowcharts*.	3. Review the data in columns 1 and 2 and identify information that needs follow-up.
Mrs. A:	Mrs. A:	Mrs. A:
Mrs. C:	Mrs. C:	Mrs. C:

It is 0800; prioritize your plan of care for both patients for the next 3 hours:

Time	Plan of Nursing Care

You return from lunch at 1200 and Mrs. A is asking for her antihypertensive medication. You know you gave the medication, but she insists that you did not give her the medication. As you investigate, the nursing assistant tells you that Mrs. C is very lethargic and unresponsive. You suddenly realize that you gave Mrs. A's 1100 medications to Mrs. C.

1. Identify the nursing interventions that you would plan to implement immediately.	2. Make a nurse's note entry as to how you might document this incident in the patient's chart/electronic medical record.

Critical reflection: To promote safe nursing practice in medication administration when caring for multiple patients, identify nursing actions:

3-10 ELDERLY PATIENT WITH MRSA

Handoff report at 11:00 PM:

"Mrs. J, 88 years old, was admitted this evening from a skilled nursing facility. The family says the patient was lethargic and confused during their visit. Her admitting vital signs were T 101° F, P 92 and irregular, R 28 and short and shallow, BP 110/70, pulse ox 94%. Her physician was called for admitting orders and was informed of the UA report from the skilled nursing facility. He will come in tomorrow morning to see her. She was given acetaminophen at 8:30 PM and her current temperature is 100.6° F; she is still slightly confused. She has an IV infusing. She is in a private room."

Mrs. J's current **flowcharts** contain the following information:

Nursing Care Kardex	Nurse's Notes from Skilled Nursing Facility
VS q4h Diet: DAT LBM: On admission IV: 0.9% NS at 75 mL/hr #24 angiocath RFA Lab: CBC, chem panel, UA **PRN Medication:** Acetaminophen 325 mg tabs ii q4h prn temp greater than 101° F	**Documentation of latest nurse's notes:** 1600 Turned, incontinent of urine, strong urine odor, incontinent pad applied. ——— ——————————————— *A. Cann LVN* 1700 Family in to visit. Upset, called physician. ——————— *A. Cann LVN* 1830 Transferred to hospital per order. Recent UA culture reports show + MRSA. Unable to contact physician to inform. Copy of report included with transfer. ——— *T. Gage RN*

Integrated Learning Activity: With a partner, **use the clinical situation and the flowcharts** to:

1. Identify the pertinent patient information made known to you in the *report*.	2. Identify the pertinent patient information made known to you in the *flowcharts*.	3. Review the data in columns 1 and 2 and identify information that needs follow-up.

It is 11:30 PM; prioritize your plan of care for the next hour:

Time	Plan of Nursing Care

Mrs. J slept 1 to 2 hours at a time during the night and remains confused. She has developed a productive cough and is expectorating a small amount of thick, creamy, yellow-colored phlegm. Her morning vital signs are T 100.8° F, P 110, R 32, BP 114/82, pulse ox 92%. At 6:30 AM the physician visits and leaves the following orders:

    Vancomycin 500 mg q8h IVPB
    Insert indwelling urinary catheter
    Bed rest
    Chest x-ray/ECG
    Oxygen 2 L/min/NP, pulse oximeter q4h
    I & O, enc. fluid intake

1. Identify the nursing interventions that you would plan to implement immediately.	2. Identify the instructions you would give to staff and family in caring for Mrs. J.

Critical reflection: To provide patient-centered care, identify nursing interventions that support the patient and family during this time:

3-11 PATIENT WITH VIRAL HEPATITIS

Handoff report at 11:00 PM:

"The patient is 27 years old and was admitted this evening. He has been diagnosed with viral hepatitis. He is very jaundiced and his urine is very dark yellow. Intake for the shift was 100 mL and output 300 mL. He does not want to eat. He says he has not had an appetite for several days. The IV was started at 5:00 PM and is on time. His 8:00 PM vital signs are T 37.5° C, P 88, R 24, BP 130/70, pain level 1, pulse ox 98%. He is currently complaining of itching and nausea and I have not medicated him. The lab reports just arrived and I put them in the patient's chart for the physician to see in the morning."

The patient's current **flowcharts** contain the following information:

Nursing Care Kardex	
VS: q4h	Diet: DAT
Bedrest c̄ BRP	
Weigh daily ☑	I & O
IV: D5/0.9 NS @125 mL/hr RFA # 22 g	
Stool for occult blood ☐	
PRN Medication: Diphenhydramine 50 mg capsule i q6h prn itching Metoclopramide 10 mg IM q6h prn N/V	

Current Lab Data
AST 460 units/L
ALT 800 units/L
Alk Phosphatase 200 units/L
Hgb 12.0 g/dL
Hct 36%
WBC 10,000/mm^3
BS 160 mg/dL
PT 24 sec (Pt. control 12-16 secs)
Total bilirubin 14 mg/dL

Integrated Learning Activity: With a partner, **use the clinical situation and the flowcharts** to:

1. Identify the pertinent patient information made known to you in the *report*.	2. Identify the pertinent patient information made known to you in the *flowcharts*.	3. Review the data in columns 1 and 2 and identify information that needs follow-up.

It is 11:30 PM; prioritize your plan of care for the next hour:

Time	Plan of Nursing Care

The patient is diagnosed with hepatitis A and is tentatively scheduled for discharge in 2 days.

---

1. Identify the discharge information that you would include in teaching the patient and his family how best to recover from hepatitis A.

Diet:	Activity:
Fluids:	Skin care:
Nausea/vomiting:	
	Sexual concerns:
Preventing transmission:	
	Alcohol intake:
	Follow-up care:

Critical reflection: To support patient-centered care and advocate teamwork and collaboration, write how you would discuss with the physician the IM order of metoclopramide:

_____

_____

_____

_____

_____

3-12 PATIENT WITH PROSTATE CANCER AND MEDICATION ERROR

Handoff report at 7:00 AM:

"Mr. T, 67 years old, has prostate cancer with metastasis to the bone. I have given him meperidine IVP around the clock for pain, the last dose given at 5:00 AM. He is lethargic but responds when spoken to. He moans periodically and is mouth breathing so he needs frequent mouth care. His urine is amber. The 6:00 AM vital signs are stable at T 99° F, P 76, R 18, BP 126/74. Intake is 100 mL, output is 150 mL. His wife spent the night in the room and is making arrangements for hospice care."

Mr. T's current **flowcharts** contain the following information:

Nursing Care Kardex	
VS: q4h	Diet: Soft
Bed rest	
Saline lock ☑	I & O
RFA # 22 g	
Urinary catheter ☑	
PRN Medication:	
Meperidine 100 mg q3h IVP prn pain	
Allergies: Morphine sulfate	
Pt: Mr. T	DNR

Physician Progress Notes

Hosp. day #3

Assess: Skin warm, dry. T 99° F
↓ oral intake
Output amber urine <600 mL/24 hr
Resp. diminished bilaterally
Alkaline phosphatase ↑
Acid phosphatase ↑

Plan: Keep comfortable
Hospice care being arranged
DNR

Integrated Learning Activity: With a partner, **use the clinical situation and the flowcharts** to:

1. Identify the pertinent patient information made known to you in the *report*.	2. Identify the pertinent patient information made known to you in the *flowcharts*.	3. Review the data in columns 1 and 2 and identify information that needs follow-up.

It is 7:30 AM; prioritize your plan of care for the next hour:

Time	Plan of Nursing Care

2:00 PM: Mrs. T calls to inform you that Mr. T is in a lot of pain and she is very upset and tells you that the pain shots do not seem to be giving him any comfort. You call the physician and suggest an order for something stronger. The physician orders morphine sulfate 15 mg IVP q3h prn pain. You administer the first dose at 2:15 PM. At 2:30 PM Mrs. T calls you into the room and tells you that her husband is not breathing. On assessment, you note that Mr. T has stopped breathing and there is no pulse.

1. Identify the nursing interventions that require immediate follow-up.	2. Identify and discuss the ethical issue presented in this situation.

Critical reflection: To promote teamwork and collaboration, identify nursing interventions that would be beneficial for you and the family at this time:

_____

_____

_____

_____

_____

_____

_____

3-13 PATIENT WITH MASTECTOMY AND IV FLUID OVERLOAD

Handoff report at 7:00 AM:

"Mrs. S, 58 years old, is 1 day postop right radical mastectomy. Her dressing is clean and dry. She has a HemoVac that drained 50 mL. Her vital signs at 6:00 AM are T 99.6° F, P 88, R 24, BP 150/90, pain level 3/10, pulse ox 95%. She is using the PCA and also has lactated Ringer's at 125 mL/hr. I started a new liter at 6:00 AM. Her right arm is elevated on a pillow; there is some swelling and she is complaining of some numbness."

Mrs. S's current **flowcharts** contain the following information:

Nursing Care Kardex	
VS: q4h	Diet: Clear liquid
Up in chair	I & O
IV: Lactated Ringer's @ 125 mL/hr	
LFA # 18 g	HemoVac ☑
Hgb & Hct this AM ☑	
Routine Medications:	
Tenormin 50 mg po bid 0900 - 1700	
PRN Medications:	
PCA with morphine sulfate at 1 mg/8 min/pt.	
demand; not to exceed 30 mg in 4 hours	

History and Physical
The patient is a 58-year-old female, widow.
She lives alone. Does not smoke, drinks socially.
Has hypertension 154/96.
Meds: Tenormin 50 mg po bid
Both parents deceased: mother died of breast cancer, father died of heart disease.
Patient has two married daughters and one son.
She found a hard lump in the right breast 3 weeks ago. A biopsy was done → Stage II CEA 5 ng/mL.

Plan: Right radical mastectomy
        Chemotherapy to follow

Integrated Learning Activity: With a partner, **use the clinical situation and the flowcharts** to:

1. Identify the pertinent patient information made known to you in the *report*.	2. Identify the pertinent patient information made known to you in the *flowcharts*.	3. Review the data in columns 1 and 2 and identify information that needs follow-up.

1.——
2.——
3.——

It is 7:30 AM; prioritize your plan of care for the next hour:

Time	Plan of Nursing Care

8:00 AM: You assess the following on Mrs. S: Alert and oriented ×4. VS: T 99° F, P 94, R 28, BP 160/100. Lung sounds with crackles in the lower bases. Surgical dressing is clean and dry. HemoVac is compressed with 10 mL of reddish drainage. Right arm is elevated on a pillow. Finger puffy, c/o of a "numbness sensation." Stated on a 0-10 pain scale, the pain level is at 2. Abdominal sounds present ×4. Antiembolic hose on. Lactated Ringer's infusing, IV site without redness or swelling, 500 mL left.

1. Identify the nursing interventions that require immediate follow-up.	2. Identify and discuss the postop educational needs of the patient.

Critical reflection: To provide patient-centered care, identify nursing interventions that would assist the patient in discussing the loss of her breast:

_____

_____

_____

_____

3-14 PATIENT WITH HF AND DIGOXIN TOXICITY

Handoff report at 7:00 AM:

"Mr. S was admitted 2 days ago with congestive heart failure. He had a restless night with some dyspnea and a dry nonproductive cough most of the night. Crackles are heard in both lungs. He has 3+ pitting edema in both legs and sacrum. His 6:00 AM vital signs are T 97.6° F, P 110 and irregular, R 34, BP 150/100, pulse ox 94% with oxygen @ 3 L/min/NC. His IV site looks slightly puffy, but there is a good blood return. He denies pain but just started to complain of nausea. His serum K$^+$ this morning is 3.0 mEq. It might be low because he is retaining fluid. His physician always comes in early so I posted the results in front of the patient's chart."

Mr. S's current **flowcharts** contain the following information:

Nursing Care Kardex

VS: q4h	Diet: 2 g Na$^+$
↑ HOB	I & O
Bed rest with BRP	
Weigh daily ☑	
O$_2$ at 3 L/min/nasal cannula	
LBM (2 days ago)	

IV: D5/0.45 NS c̄ 20 mEq KCl q12h
L hand # 20 g

LAB:
Digoxin level ☑
K$^+$, Na$^+$, BUN, creatinine, AST ☑

DX: CHF	Age: 72

Medication Record

Routine	Time
Digoxin 0.25 mg po qAM	0900
Furosemide 40 mg IVP BID	0900 - 1700
K-Dur 10 mEq po BID	0900 - 1700
Captopril 6.25 mg po TID	0900 - 1700 - 2200
Colace 100 mg po qAM	0900

PRN

NTG SL 0.4 mg tab i q5min x3 doses prn chest pain

THREE

Integrated Learning Activity: With a partner, **use the clinical situation and the flowcharts** to:

1. Identify the pertinent patient information made known to you in the *report*.	2. Identify the pertinent patient information made known to you in the *flowcharts*.	3. Review the data in columns 1 and 2 and identify information that needs follow-up.

It is 7:30 AM; prioritize your plan of care for the next hour:

Time	Plan of Nursing Care

9:00 AM: The physician has not come in to see Mr. S. Mr. S is alert but experiencing increasing shortness of breath, cough, and nausea and complaining of blurred vision. His pulse oximetry result is 88%. P 116 and irregular, R 34 and short and shallow, BP 152/100. Skin cool, color with slight cyanosis. Aside from the K^+ of 3.0 mEq, Mr. S's Na^+ is 135+ mEq, and his digoxin level is 2.4 ng/mL. You call the physician and learn that he is in surgery and will call you back within 30 minutes.

1. Identify the nursing interventions that require immediate follow-up.	2. Write a nurse's note to describe the 9:00 AM situation and the follow-up interventions.

Critical reflection: To provide safe nursing care, identify how clinical reasoning was used to make a clinical decision.

3-15 PATIENT WITH HIP FRACTURE AND DVT

Handoff report at 7:00 AM:

"Mrs. LV, 74 years old, is 4 days postop left hip fracture. She had a ConstaVac that was removed yesterday. Surgical dressing is clean and dry. Pedal pulse on the left foot is present and the circulation, movement, and sensation are within normal limits. Lung sounds with fine crackles at the lower bases in both lungs. You need to encourage her to deep breathe and use the incentive spirometer. Her 6:00 AM vital signs are T 99.8° F, P 80, R 18, BP 130/82, pulse ox 96%. She does not want to move, it seems like she is scared. I have given her acetaminophen #3 two times during the night for leg pain, the last dose was at 6:00 AM. She is sleeping right now."

Mrs. LV's current **flowcharts** contain the following information:

Nursing Care Kardex

VS: q shift   Diet: Soft
HOH   I & O
Ambulate with PT
LBM (2 days ago)
IV: Saline lock LFA #22 g angiocath
       Inserted day of surgery

Routine Medications:

Digoxin 0.125 mg po qAM   0900
Furosemide 10 mg po qAM   0900
FeSO$_4$ 300 mg po tid c̄ meals 0800 - 1200 - 1700
Lovenox 30 mg subcut daily   0900

PRN:

Acetaminophen with codeine #3 tab i po q4h prn pain

Medical History

Elderly female brought into the ED after falling at home. A fracture of the left hip was diagnosed. She was taken to surgery and an ORIF was performed.

Hgb 9.4 mg/dL, Hct 28% on admission.

Patient has a history of atrial fibrillation.

She lives alone, has one son, and her husband died 2 years ago from a cardiac condition.

Integrated Learning Activity: With a partner, **use the clinical situation and the flowcharts** to:

1. Identify the pertinent patient information made known to you in the *report*.	2. Identify the pertinent patient information made known to you in the *flowcharts*.	3. Review the data in columns 1 and 2 and identify information that needs follow-up.

It is 7:30 AM; prioritize your plan of care for the next hour:

Time	Plan of Nursing Care

You review the nurse's notes from the night shift and note the following:

12:00 AM   Alert, moaning, states leg hurts, pain level 7. Circulation, movement, and sensation of left leg WNL. Dressing clean and dry. Repositioned. Acetaminophen with codeine #3 tab i given for pain.

2:00 AM   Awake, states pain in leg, does not want to be touched. Left pedal pulse palpable. Repositioned.

4:00 AM   Sleeping.

6:00 AM   c/o leg pain, pain level remains at 7. Medicated with acetaminophen with codeine #3 tab i given for pain.

You enter the following assessment in the nurse's notes:

7:30 AM Awake, alert, states "did not have a good night." Right leg pain level at 5. Left leg with pedal pulse, warm, cap. refill greater than 2 sec. Leg elevated on pillow. Dressing clean and dry. Right leg with weak pedal pulse, swelling and redness noted at calf and thigh. Tender to touch. Lung sounds with fine crackles, encouraged to take deep breaths. Bowel sounds present ×4, complaining of constipation.

DVT

1. Identify the nursing interventions that require immediate follow-up.	2. Identify the instructions that you will give the nursing assistants at this time.
	have vitals checked

Critical reflection: To promote safe nursing practice, the handoff report at 7:00 AM:

☐ communicated sufficient information to provide continuous care to the patient.

☐ lacked the following: _____

3-16 PATIENT DIAGNOSED WITH PULMONARY EMBOLUS AND ON ANTICOAGULANT THERAPY

Handoff report at 3:00 PM:

"Mrs. L was admitted with signs and symptoms of having developed a pulmonary embolus. She just had a baby 2 weeks ago. She has a heparin drip. The infusion pump is set at 20 mL/hr. You have 100 mL left. She slept well. Respirations are unlabored at 22. The right lower lung has diminished breath sounds. She will be started on Coumadin today. She is anxious to go home and be with her baby."

Mrs. L's current **flowcharts** contain the following information:

Nursing Care Kardex

VS: q4h   Diet: Regular

Bed rest with BRP   I & O
O₂ @ 3 L/min/NC prn SOB

IV: 500 mL D5W c̄ 20,000 units heparin
    Infuse at 1000 units/hr
    LFA #22 g angiocath

LAB:
Daily PTT ☑ PT in AM

Routine Medications:
Coumadin 5 mg po today at 0900
Coumadin 2.5 mg po today at 1700

Coagulation Record

Date	PTT	Control	Heparin dose
1st day	50 sec	25 sec	900 units/hr
2nd day	60 sec	25 sec	1000 units/hr
3rd day	90 sec	30 sec	1100 units/hr
Current	75 sec	30 sec	1000 units/hr

Integrated Learning Activity: With a partner, **use the clinical situation and the flowcharts** to:

1. Identify the pertinent patient information made known to you in the *report*.	2. Identify the pertinent patient information made known to you in the *flowcharts*.	3. Review the data in columns 1 and 2 and identify information that needs follow-up.

It is 3:30 PM; prioritize your plan of care for the next hour:

Time	Plan of Nursing Care

6:30 PM The nursing assistant informs you that the IV pump is beeping. You go into assess the pump and you notice that the heparin bag is empty. You look at the infusion pump and it is set at 35 mL/hr instead of 25 mL/hr.

1. **Identify the nursing interventions that require immediate follow-up.**	2. **Document your findings as you would enter them in the nursing notes.**

Critical reflection: To promote safe nursing practice, identify interventions that support the safe administration of heparin therapy and professional competency:

3-17 PATIENT WITH SIGNS AND SYMPTOMS OF POSTOP COMPLICATIONS

Handoff report at 3:00 PM:

"Ms. P, 23 years old, had an emergency appendectomy yesterday. She has Down syndrome. She has gotten up to the chair twice today. Surgical dressing is clean, dry, and intact. Bowel sounds are hypoactive. Her IV is infusing well; you have 200 mL left. Oral intake is 100 mL and output is 400 mL. I gave her morphine sulfate 8 mg IVP at noon for pain. Her noon vital signs are T 100° F, P 80, R 20, BP 110/78, pulse ox 98%."

Ms. P's current **flowcharts** contain the following information:

Nursing Care Kardex	
VS: q4h	Diet: Clear liquid
Ambulate c̄ assistance	I & O
IV: IL D5/0.9% NS @ 125 mL/hr LFA #22 g angiocath	
Routine Medications: Cefoxitin 1 g IVPB q8h 1000 - 1800 - 0200	
PRN Medications: Morphine sulfate 8 mg IVP q4h prn pain Droperidol 1.25 mg IVP q4h prn N/V	

Intake and Output Record

7 – 3 shift:

Oral:	100	Void:	8:00 AM	50
			9:00	50
			11:00	75
			12:00	50
			1:00 PM	75
IV:	900		2:00	100
IVPB:	50			
		Emesis	12:00 PM	100
Total:	1050		Total:	500

Integrated Learning Activity: With a partner, **use the clinical situation and the flowcharts** to:

1. Identify the pertinent patient information made known to you in the *report*.	2. Identify the pertinent patient information made known to you in the *flowcharts*.	3. Review the data in columns 1 and 2 and identify information that needs follow-up.

THREE

It is 3:30 PM; prioritize your plan of care for the next hour:

Time	Plan of Nursing Care

8:00 PM: Ms. P's mother and family are at the bedside. They tell you that Ms. P is increasingly restless and is pulling at her surgical dressing. You note the following entries in the nursing notes:
Has voided a total of 100 mL since 4:00 PM. Emesis 100 mL greenish fluid at 6:00 PM, refused dinner.
Morphine sulfate 8 mg and droperidol 1.25 mg given IVP at 6:00 PM.

1. Identify the nursing interventions that require immediate follow-up.	2. Identify a rationale for each nursing intervention that you plan to implement.

Critical reflection: To provide patient-centered care, identify nursing interventions that support the patient and family during this time:

3-18 PATIENT WITH CELLULITIS DEVELOPS ANGINA

Handoff report at 0700:

"Mr. O has cellulitis of the right leg. He is pretty much self-care and he says he is not used to being in bed so much. He stays in a chair most of the time with his leg elevated. His I & O is fine and his vital signs are stable at T 37° C, P 92, R 22, BP 164/94, pain level 0, pulse ox 98%. He has a dry dressing on the right leg and there is no drainage. His saline lock needs to be changed today and his fingerstick blood glucose was 110 this morning."

Mr. O's current **flowcharts** contain the following information:

Nursing Care Kardex
VS: q4h   Diet: 2000 cal ADA
BRP
4x4 to right leg - Change q shift
LBM 1 day ago   I & O
IV: Saline lock
LFA #22 g angiocath
O₂ @ 3 L/min/NP prn
Elevate leg on pillow
Fingerstick BG qAM   0600 ☑
Mr. O   62 yr   Dx: Cellulitis R. Leg
Hx: Angina, hypertension, DM type 2

O_2 @ 3 L/min/NP prn

Medication Administration Record		
Routine meds:		
Glyburide 10 mg po qAM	0800	
Verapamil SR 240 mg po bid	0900	1700
Propranolol 20 mg po bid	0900	1700
ASA 81 mg po qAM	0900	
Colace 100 mg po qAM	0900	
Cephradine 2 g IVPB q6h	2400-0600-	
	1200-1800	
PRN:		
NTG SL 0.4 mg q5min ×3 prn chest pain		

Integrated Learning Activity: With a partner, **use the clinical situation and the flowcharts** to:

1. Identify the pertinent patient information made known to you in the *report*.	2. Identify the pertinent patient information made known to you in the *flowcharts*.	3. Review the data in columns 1 and 2 and identify information that needs follow-up.

It is 0730; prioritize your plan of care for the next hour:

Time	Plan of Nursing Care

1200: Mr. O returns to bed after having a BM. You note that he is short of breath and his skin is cool and clammy. You assess his vital signs, his radial pulse is 110 and irregular, respirations are 32, and his BP is 170/100. He tells you that he is feeling pressure on his chest. You assist him into bed and place him in high Fowler position.

1. Identify your follow-up nursing interventions.	2. Identify a rationale for each nursing intervention that you plan to implement.

Critical reflection: To provide patient-centered care, identify nursing interventions that support the patient and family during this time:

3-19 PATIENT WITH TURP AND NS IRRIGATION

Handoff report at 7:00 AM:

"Mr. I, 70 years old, is 1 day postop TURP. He has a continuous normal saline irrigation. I will hang up a new irrigation bag before I leave. He has had several clots during the shift. His vital signs are T 37.2° C, P 90, R 22, BP 160/93. He is alert and cheerful, and told me that he leads a very active life. I gave him a suppository for c/o bladder spasms at 5 this morning for a pain level of 7 out of 10. The IV was started at 1:00 AM and it is behind since it slows down when the patient bends his arm."

Mr. I's current **flowcharts** contain the following information:

Nursing Care Rand

VS q4h   Diet: Soft diet
Antiembolic hose on
LBM: On admission
IV: Lactated Ringer's at 75 mL/hr
#20 g angiocath RFA

3-way indwelling cath c̄ 30-mL balloon
NS cont irrigation - keep UA free of clots
Manual bladder irrigation with NS prn

Routine Medication:
Colace 100 mg po qAM   1000
PRN Medication:
B & O supp. i q6h prn bladder spasms

Intake and Output Record

11-7 shift:

	Intake	Output
Oral:	50	1300
		(NS irrigation 1000)
IV:	300	
Total:	350 mL	300 mL

Integrated Learning Activity: With a partner, **use the clinical situation and the flowcharts** to:

1. Identify the pertinent patient information made known to you in the *report*.	2. Identify the pertinent patient information made known to you in the *flowcharts*.	3. Review the data in columns 1 and 2 and identify information that needs follow-up.

It is 7:30 AM; prioritize your plan of care for the next hour:

Time	Plan of Nursing Care

8:00 AM: Mr. I is complaining of increased pain. He is grimacing, is diaphoretic, and tells you he has an urge to urinate. You note that the irrigation bag is empty and there are 50 mL of burgundy-colored urine in the urinary collection bag. There is urine leaking around the catheter.

1. Identify the nursing interventions that you would plan to implement immediately.	2. Identify the follow-up nursing interventions for the rest of the shift.

Critical reflection: To promote safe nursing practice, the handoff report at 7:00 AM and the flowcharts:

☐ communicated sufficient information to provide continuous care to the patient.

☐ lacked the following: _____

_____

_____

_____

_____

_____

3-20 PATIENT WITH TAH AND EPIDURAL CATHETER

Handoff report at 7:00 AM:

"Mrs. F, 46 years old, had a TAH-BSO yesterday. She had soft bowel sounds this morning. The abdominal dressing is clean and dry. Her peripheral IV is infusing well and she has an epidural infusion with fentanyl infusing through a pump. She has not had any breakthrough pain. The epidural dressing is intact and the catheter is fine. She has been mostly on bed rest, but she is to get up to a chair this morning. The 6:00 AM vital signs are T 37.5° C, P 78, R 18, BP 130/80, pulse ox 98%. Her output was 500 mL."

Mrs. F's current **flowcharts** contain the following information:

Nursing Care Rand

VS: q4h   Diet: Clear liquids

Up in chair with assistance
Incentive spirometer q1h ×10 while awake
LBM: Prior to admission

Urinary catheter ☑

IV: D5/0.45% NS q8h LFA 20 g angiocath

Routine Medication:
Fentanyl infusion @ 6 mL/hr/pump via epidural catheter ordered by anesthesiologist

Intake and Output Record

Night shift:

Intake		Output	
Oral: (Sips of H_2O)	50	Void:	
		UA cath:	500
IV:	1000		
IV (fentanyl):	48		

⚡ **Integrated Learning Activity:** With a partner, **use the clinical situation and the flowcharts** to:

1. Identify the pertinent patient information made known to you in the *report*.	2. Identify the pertinent patient information made known to you in the *flowcharts*.	3. Review the data in columns 1 and 2 and identify information that needs follow-up.

It is 7:30 AM; prioritize your plan of care for the next hour:

Time	Plan of Nursing Care

At 8:30 AM: Mrs. F gets up with assistance to sit in a chair. As she walks slowly to the chair, she steps on some of the tubing. The nursing assistant tells you that the infusion pump is beeping. You go in to assess and note that the infusion pump is beeping and the patient's epidural dressing is pulled from the patient's back. The epidural catheter is pulled out.

1. Identify the nursing interventions that you would plan to implement immediately.	2. Document your findings as you would enter them in the nursing notes.

Critical reflection: To provide patient-centered care, identify nursing interventions that support the patient during this time:

_____

_____

_____

_____

_____

3-21 CULTURALLY COMPETENT NURSING CARE

The nurse reviews the history and physical (H & P) and the care plan of the assigned patient:

Admitting Information: Mr. W, 72-year-old male of Chinese descent. Brought into the office by his son. The son provided most of the information because the patient speaks limited English. The patient lives in China but has been in the U.S. for 5 months visiting his son. He was planning to return home in a couple of weeks. Mr. W requests that the son be present and assist with questions during his physical exam.

Physical Examination:

Appearance: Small frame, thin man.

VS: T 101.8° F, P 92, R 28, BP 130/90, pulse oximetry 94%

Neuro: Alert, soft-spoken, smiles and answers questions appropriately via the son. PERRLA.

Resp: Crackles bilaterally. Productive cough with yellow-colored phlegm. Dyspnea. Indicates that "chest hurts all over."

CV: Pulse slightly irregular. Murmur—neg.

Integ: Dry, decreased turgor.

GI: Abdomen soft, nontender. Son states his father is not eating very well. He misses the traditional cooking but does like some American soups. Denies constipation.

GU: No complaints. WNL.

Psychosocial: Quiet, widower.

Medications: Prescription medications—none. Has been using several herbal teas for "the cold in his chest."

Admitting Dx: Bilateral Pneumonia

Day Shift Report to Evening Shift: Mr. W has been in the hospital for 2 days. There is always someone in the room with the patient. His son spent the night with him.

The patient is quiet and speaks limited English. He seems to respond better to male nurses. Lung sounds are still diminished in the lower bases. Has refused his bath for 2 days now. He has lost another pound since admission. His IV is infusing well at 125 mL/hr and Cefizox IVPB is ordered q12h.

Day Shift Nursing Notes:

0800 Neuro: Awake, quiet, and cooperative. PERRLA.

Resp: Diminished in the lower bilateral bases. Productive cough with light yellowish sputum. Pulse ox 94%. O_2 at 2 L/min/NC. SOB noted on exertion.

CV/Skin: Warm, cap refill less than 3 sec. Turgor nonelastic.

GI: Active bowel sounds ×4 quadrants.--N. Nurse RN

0900 GI: Ate 50% of breakfast. Family has brought in some food for the patient.

MS: Up to bathroom with assistance from the son. SOB noted on exertion. Son states that the father is upset because he believes his urine smells bad because of the IV medication.---------- N. Nurse RN

1300 GI: Ate 10% of lunch. Drinking teas and soups brought from home.-------------- N. Nurse RN

1400 Systems unchanged. ----------------N. Nurse RN

Integrated Learning Activity: With a partner, **use the clinical situation and the flowcharts** to:

1. Identify the pertinent patient information made known to you in the *report*.	2. Identify the pertinent patient information made known to you in the *flowcharts*.	3. Review the data in columns 1 and 2 and identify information that needs follow-up.

Use the **Cultural Considerations** listed in the left-hand side of the following box to develop **realistic nursing interventions** that demonstrate culturally sensitive care for Mr. W:

Cultural Considerations	Care Plan
• Communication • Food preferences • View of health care practitioner role • Patient's role in the family • Patient's view of Western medicine with regard to current illness • Patient's view of what caused the illness • Patient's view of what would be beneficial for getting better	

On the third hospital day, Mr. W refuses the morning dose of Cefizox IVPB and refuses to let the nurse listen to his lungs. He tells the family that he is tired and wants to be left alone. His 0800 VS are T 99.9° F, P 96, R 26, BP 134/90, pulse oximetry 86%.

1. Identify the nursing interventions that you would implement at this time.	2. Identify a rationale for each intervention that you plan to implement.

Critical reflection: To provide patient-centered care, identify nursing interventions that support the patient and family during this time:

_____

_____

_____

_____

_____

_____

3-22 PATIENT WITH ANTHRAX EXPOSURE

Mr. S, 46 years old, comes into the urgent care center with complaints of fatigue, muscle aches, a cough, and headache. Vital signs are T 99.8° F, P 90, R 28, BP 130/88. Mr. S tells the nurse that he has had these symptoms for the last 48 hours and that he cannot afford to be ill. He says that he has a lot of work waiting for him at the office because there have been rumors regarding anthrax exposure of several people from one of the government buildings several blocks away.

The information obtained from Mr. S includes:

Examination	Familial History	Social History
Neuro: A & O c/o slight headache. Resp: Bilateral wheezing. Non-productive cough, SOB noted. c/o sore throat and chest area "a little sore." CV: Regular pulse, heart sounds WNL GI: Anorexia. Abdomen soft, nontender. GU: WNL	Married, 2 children, both healthy (1 male, 15 years; 1 female, 12 years). Wife works as a secretary part-time. Mother: Deceased; trauma from an auto accident. Father: DM type 2, hypertension. **Employment History:** Government employee for 15 years.	Alcohol: Drinks occasionally. Medications: Vitamins, echinacea tablets (heard it helped in decreasing the effects of a cold). Activities: Golfs twice a month, gym (weights and treadmill). Describes himself as a "generally healthy person."

Integrated Learning Activity: With a partner, **use the clinical situation and the information obtained** to:

1. Identify the pertinent patient information made known to you in the *report*.	2. Identify the pertinent patient information made known to you in the *flowcharts*.	3. Review the data in columns 1 and 2 and identify information that needs follow-up.

THREE

The patient is diagnosed and admitted to the acute-care setting with signs and symptoms of inhalation anthrax. Read the following **physician orders** and **write a rationale** for each order:

Physician Orders	
Physician Orders 1. Standard precautions 2. Chest x-ray stat 3. VS q4h with neuro checks 4. CBC, 12-chem panel, UA 5. Ciprofloxacin 400 mg IVPB now	**1. Standard precautions:** _____ _____ **2. Chest x-ray stat:** _____ _____ **3. VS q4h with neuro checks:** _____ **4. CBC, 12-chem panel, UA:** _____ **5. Ciprofloxacin 400 mg IVPB now:** _____

At 1600 the nursing assistant reports the following: T 99° F, P 120, R 30, BP 118/80, pulse oximetry 92%. The patient was difficult to arouse.

1. Identify the nursing interventions that you would plan to implement immediately.	2. Identify a rationale for each nursing intervention that you plan to implement.

Critical reflection: To provide patient-centered care, identify nursing interventions that support the patient and family during this time:

_____

_____

_____

_____

4-1 MENTORING AND NURSING MANAGEMENT

The supervisor of a medical unit has recently hired several new RNs just out of nursing school. Two of the new RNs have started on the day shift. As an RN with 7 years of experience, you have been assigned to orient and precept one of the new RNs. The new RN will work with you for 3 months.

Information about the experienced RN: You have worked mainly on the medical unit and are considered an expert. You are always on time. You are organized and can be counted on "to get the job done." You are frequently given all the new employees to orient. You have never complained and you like working with nurses, but you are getting pretty tired of having to be the one that is assigned to orient the new employees all the time.

Information about the new RN: He is in his twenties, quiet but friendly. He works steadily, has a good knowledge base, but has difficulty asking questions. He has managed the care of three patients in school. He was late the first day on the unit and tells the nurse that he "is more of a night person."

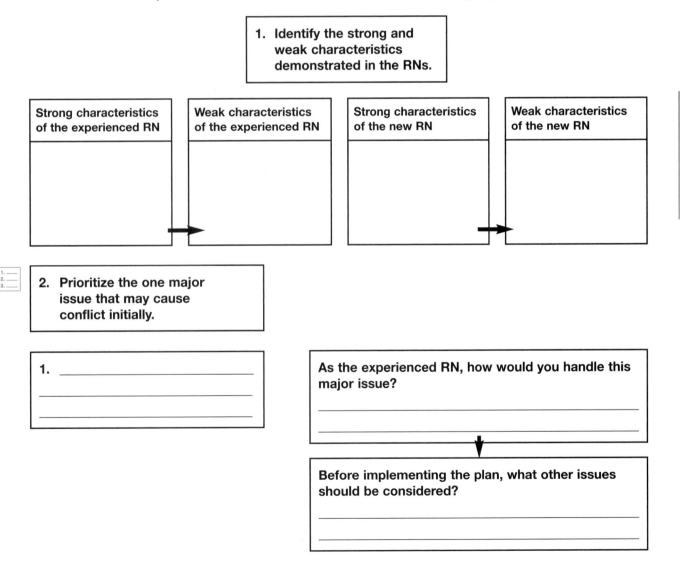

1. **Identify the strong and weak characteristics demonstrated in the RNs.**

Strong characteristics of the experienced RN	Weak characteristics of the experienced RN	Strong characteristics of the new RN	Weak characteristics of the new RN

2. **Prioritize the one major issue that may cause conflict initially.**

1. _____
   _____
   _____

As the experienced RN, how would you handle this major issue?
_____
_____

Before implementing the plan, what other issues should be considered?
_____
_____

FOUR

As the experienced nurse, you develop the following goals to help guide the progress of the new RN. You discuss these goals with the new RN.

Goals for the First Week	Goals for the Second Week

At the end of the 2 weeks, the new RN has not been able to achieve the set goals. The experienced RN sets up a time to meet with the new RN. During the meeting, the new RN is visibly upset.

> 1. Identify the issues that may be affecting the new RN

Issues:

_____
_____
_____
_____
_____
_____

With a partner, role-play the part of the experienced nurse and the new RN.

As the experienced RN, how would you handle this situation?	As the new RN, how would you like this situation handled?

4-2 WORKING THROUGH THE CHANGE PROCESS

The hospital administration has decided to implement a new electronic medical record program to be used in all of the nursing units for charting patient assessments. For the last 6 months the staff has been required to attend computer training classes offered at the hospital. Training manuals and informational flyers have been placed in all the units. For months, employees have heard talk and rumors about this new change, but no one actually believed that it would happen so soon. Now the units seem chaotic as the technology staff installs the new computers while the nurses work around them to provide patient care.

Information about administration's decision: The electronic medical record program has been studied for months. Charge nurses and staff nurses from all shifts have been involved in evaluating the program and giving feedback. The administration has invested time and money into this form of charting and is committed to implementing this program throughout the hospital. Electronic medical record training was mandatory.

Information about the nursing staff: The implementation of the new charting format has brought about mixed feelings among the nursing staff. The younger nurses are excited and think that the charting will be "fun." The older nurses feel that it will take more time and do not understand how the electronic medical record program will make charting easier. Comments from nurses range from "Isn't this exciting?" to "The administration can spend thousands of dollars in these computers but has a hard time giving us a raise when we are the ones doing all the work." The managers, supervisors, and charge nurses are asked to support this change and to ensure that all nursing staff is trained.

FOUR

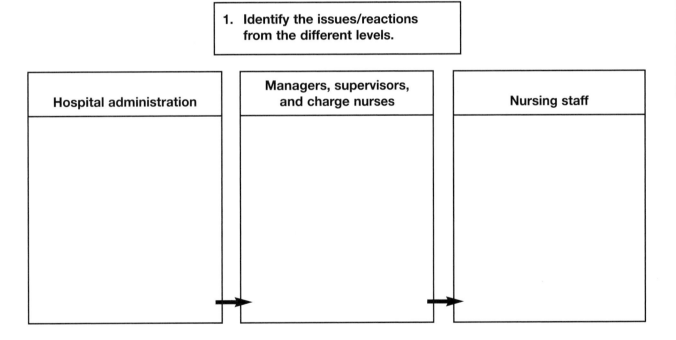

1. **Identify the issues/reactions from the different levels.**

Hospital administration	Managers, supervisors, and charge nurses	Nursing staff

How does the implementation of the electronic medical record and the nursing staff's comments and feelings correlate with the change process?

_____

_____

_____

You are the charge nurse of the unit that has been selected to be the first one to use the new computerized program. Some nurses are very excited to be the first ones to use the program and other nurses are requesting to transfer to another unit. Administration has asked you to ensure that all nursing staff use the program and to identify how the administrative staff can help you facilitate the implementation of this computerized program on your unit.

1. Identify helpful strategies that support the implementation and help your staff cope with the change.	2. Identify specific requests that can guide administration in helping you and your staff implement this change.

How does the development of **helpful strategies,** both for the nursing staff and for administration, help with the process of change?

_____

_____

_____

After 2 weeks of using the program, your most experienced nurse requests to be transferred to a unit that is not using the electronic medical record program at this time. You, as the charge nurse, know that all the units will be using the electronic medical record program within the next 6 months. The nurse is very good and you do not want to lose her.

As the charge nurse, how would you handle this situation?	As the nurse, how would you like this situation handled?

4-3 TEAMWORK AND DELEGATION

An RN is transferred to the medical unit after working 5 years in the intensive care unit. It has taken some time—3 months to be exact—to organize and manage the care of 4 to 5 patients assigned to her on the day shift. The patients on the medical unit are high acuity and have multiple problems. Most of the staff has been very supportive, always checking to see whether they can help. However, the RN has observed one nursing assistant who rarely helps out the other staff members. The RN also believes that some interventions that the nursing assistant has done have been performed incorrectly.

Information about the RN: The RN is used to working independently. She would rather do the procedure or provide the care herself to ensure that it is done correctly. This has been a difficult transition for her because she has to rely on ancillary help to complete her work. Although the RN can delegate many tasks, she finds herself avoiding this nursing assistant and mostly doing the tasks herself. She stays late everyday to complete the charting on the patients.

Information about the nursing assistant: The nursing assistant has been on this unit for 1 year. She feels pretty comfortable with her skills and has even shown other nursing assistants how to take short cuts. She enjoys working by herself and takes pride in not asking anyone for help. She does not like being told how to do something that she already knows how to do. She is frustrated with the RN because the RN seems to be running around in circles. As far as she is concerned, she will do her job, and, unless asked, she will not do anything extra.

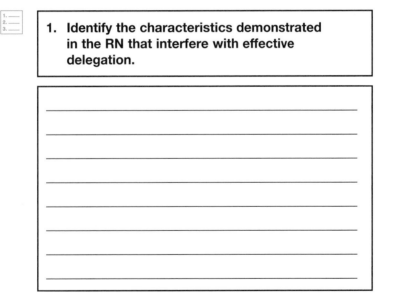

1. **Identify the characteristics demonstrated in the RN that interfere with effective delegation.**

In managing this situation, what can the RN do to create a more conducive working environment with the nursing assistant?

_____

_____

_____

The following day the nursing assistant is assigned to work with the RN. There are numerous tasks that need to be done on the patients. The nurse has the following tasks that need to be done for the assigned patients: vital signs, three bed baths, assessments, saline lock flushes, emptying urinary collection bags on two patients, emptying a J-P device, W-D dressing change, passing narcotic medications, monitoring IV fluids, NG tube bolus feeding, oral suctioning, deep suctioning, pulse oximetry, and starting oxygen per nasal cannula.

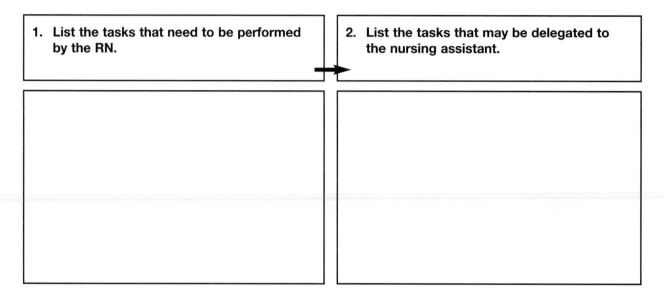

1. List the tasks that need to be performed by the RN.	2. List the tasks that may be delegated to the nursing assistant.

List the criteria that should be considered before delegating a task to another person.

_____

_____

_____

After the RN has taken her own noon vital signs, the nursing assistant approaches her and asks her why she did not let her take the noon vitals on the patients.

With a partner, role-play the part of the RN and the nursing assistant.

As the RN, how would you problem-solve this situation?	As the nursing assistant, what would you like to come out of this situation?

4-4 PRACTICE AND ETHICAL ISSUE

Two RNs have worked the day shift together on the oncology unit for several years. Both are expert nurses and through the years they have become close personal friends. RN Nurse A has accepted the position of charge nurse of the oncology unit, and RN Nurse B continues as a staff nurse. For the last 6 months, the charge nurse has been concerned about numerous discrepancies in the narcotic count. Lately, an increasing number of patients have been complaining that they are not obtaining pain relief after being medicated. After a careful investigation by the administrative staff, it was noted that all the narcotic count discrepancies occurred on the day shift. RN Nurse A, the charge nurse, is the only person informed of the current findings. A follow-up investigation will be conducted.

Information about RN Nurse A: The RN is married and has two children. She is frequently involved with the school activities of the children. She loves the staff and enjoys her work but is still learning the duties of a manager. She has a difficult time supervising and evaluating staff and seems to avoid handling any conflict situations. She has noticed that RN Nurse B has been irritable but has assumed that her recent marital separation is contributing to her behavior. After assessing the behavior of RN Nurse B, she is wondering whether her friend may be involved with the narcotic discrepancies.

Information about RN Nurse B: The RN has two children in school and has recently separated from her husband. She has been unable to be active in her children's school activities because of the added demands brought on by the separation. She has been suffering from migraine headaches but cannot afford to miss any work because the couple had just purchased a new home before the separation. She has asked RN Nurse A to assign her to extra shifts or overtime whenever possible.

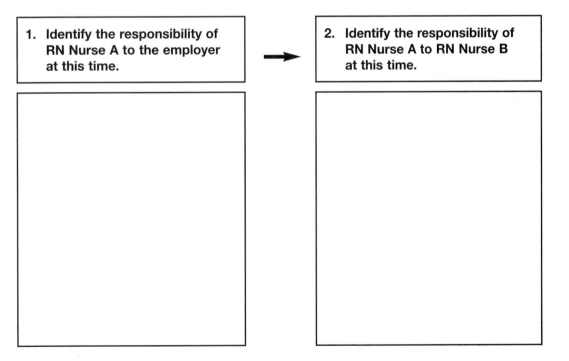

1. Identify the responsibility of RN Nurse A to the employer at this time.

2. Identify the responsibility of RN Nurse A to RN Nurse B at this time.

RN Nurse A feels that she is not being honest with the staff by not sharing the administrative decision to conduct a preliminary investigation. Identify issues that should be considered in this situation.

_____

_____

_____

FOUR

For 3 weeks the narcotic count has been correct. Today, RN Nurse B is assigned to a terminally ill patient. She is preparing to administer pain medication to a patient and takes a syringe labeled morphine sulfate 10 mg from the narcotic drawer. She administers the medication IV to the patient. Thirty minutes later the patient is moaning with pain, and the family is very upset seeing him in such pain. The physician is called, and an order for a stat dose of morphine sulfate 5 mg IV is given. RN Nurse A administers the drug to the patient because RN Nurse B is at lunch. The patient is calm for the next 2 hours. RN Nurse A informs RN Nurse B about the additional dose of pain medication given to the patient. At the end of the shift, there is a discrepancy with the morphine sulfate and the narcotic count.

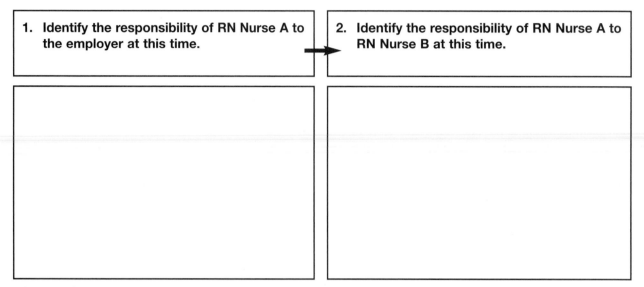

1. Identify the responsibility of RN Nurse A to the employer at this time.	2. Identify the responsibility of RN Nurse A to RN Nurse B at this time.

The next day, RN Nurse B is again preparing to administer morphine sulfate 10 mg IV push to the patient. RN Nurse B emptied the contents of the morphine sulfate into another syringe and put this syringe in her pocket. She then filled the current syringe with saline solution and took this syringe into the room and gave the saline solution to the patient.

RN Nurse A noticed that RN Nurse B had a syringe with liquid in her pocket as she was going home. RN Nurse A confronts RN Nurse B. RN Nurse B tells her friend that it is saline solution, but she refuses to discard it or to give it to RN Nurse A. With a partner, role-play the part of the RN Nurse A and the RN Nurse B.

As RN Nurse A, identify the outcome of RN Nurse B's action.	Identify the professional responsibility of RN Nurse A.

As RN Nurse B, what would you like to come out of this situation?

4-5 TEAMWORK AND COLLABORATION

The RN works on an endocrine unit in a hospital that uses a team approach to deliver patient care. The team consists of an RN, an LVN, and two nursing assistants. The RN is responsible for the supervision and the delegation of care. A new, highly recommended LVN has recently been hired to work on the unit. During the first week of orientation, the supervising RN noticed that the LVN was friendly but did not check the insulin dosages with anyone before giving the insulin injections to the patients. The RN told the LVN to have all insulin dosages double-checked before giving. The LVN told one of the nursing assistants that the RN did not trust her. Later, the RN again saw the LVN giving an insulin injection to another patient without checking the insulin dose. The RN questioned the LVN, and the LVN responded that she forgot because she never had to have her work checked in her previous job and she would remember to double-check the dose next time.

Information about the RN: The RN has been working on the endocrine unit for 2 years. She is very conscientious and, because she has diabetes mellitus, she takes a special interest in working with patients who have diabetes. She works closely with her staff and has not had any serious staff problems. She can tell that the LVN has a lot of experience and feels a little intimidated by her at times. The RN has little patience for what she considers "unsafe practice" behaviors.

Information about the LVN: The LVN has been a nurse for 15 years and is recognized for providing good patient care. She has worked in several hospitals. In her last job, she worked in a skilled nursing facility where she had increased responsibility. She decided to return to the acute care setting because it offered better financial benefits. She feels that she has a lot of experience and is more familiar with some clinical situations than the newly graduated RNs. She can tell that the staff RN is recently out of school.

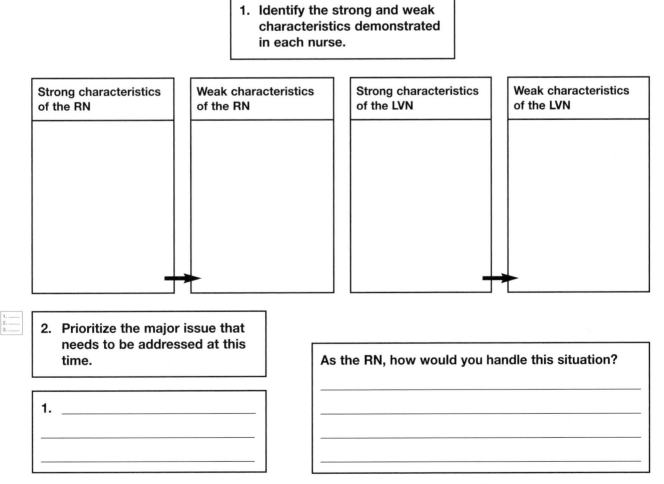

1. **Identify the strong and weak characteristics demonstrated in each nurse.**

Strong characteristics of the RN	Weak characteristics of the RN	Strong characteristics of the LVN	Weak characteristics of the LVN

2. **Prioritize the major issue that needs to be addressed at this time.**

1. _____

As the RN, how would you handle this situation?

_____

_____

_____

_____

FOUR

For the next 2 weeks, the RN noticed that the LVN had been double-checking the insulin dosages. Today, the unit is very busy and one patient in particular is very upset and requested to speak with the RN. The patient complained of several things but was especially upset because he was going to receive the wrong dose of insulin this morning. The patient explained that he asked the LVN how much insulin she was giving him and that she said 10 units of Humulin N. The patient insisted that he normally was given 12 units of Humulin N every morning. The LVN checked and the patient was correct.

The RN discussed the patient's comments with the LVN. The LVN agreed with the patient's comments, telling the RN that because the 10 units of Humulin N was less than the ordered dose, it was easily corrected. The RN decided to set up a meeting with the LVN to discuss the incident further and to present the following anecdotal note:

12/31 0900 Patient X complained that the LVN was going to administer 10 units of Humulin N insulin to him this morning instead of the ordered Humulin N 12 units. The LVN rechecked the ordered amount and proceeded to administer the correct dose to the patient.

I have told the LVN to double-check all insulin dosages before administering the injection to the patients. The LVN does not realize the seriousness of this behavior.

Discuss, evaluate, and rewrite the anecdotal note.

Anecdotal notes should contain:

The RN meets with the LVN.

With a partner, role-play the part of the RN and the LVN.

As the RN, how would you handle this situation?

_____

_____

_____

_____

_____

_____

_____

_____

Identify key points to keep in mind when conducting an evaluation meeting with an employee.

_____

_____

_____

_____

_____

_____

_____

4-6 ADVOCATING CULTURAL COMPETENCY AND SENSITIVITY

The medical unit staff of an acute care hospital includes several RNs who have worked on this unit for more than 10 years. In addition to caring for high-acuity patients, the nurses on the medical unit have also seen a change in the cultural makeup of the staff. The hospital has recently hired six new RNs from various ethnic backgrounds: two Middle Eastern nurses, one Chinese nurse, one Korean nurse, one Hispanic nurse, and one male nurse from Nigeria. All the nurses were trained outside the United States and were successful in passing the NCLEX-RN examination. Although all the nurses have taken additional classes and training, this is their first full-time job in the acute-care setting.

After going through the regular hospital orientation, the nurses are assigned to work on the day and evening shifts. After 2 months, three of the female nurses are having great difficulty working on the medical unit. Several of the regular RNs are complaining that the new nurses are not as competent and that they do not know how to relate with the staff and with the patients. Several staff members have asked to be transferred to another unit.

The unit manager solicited input from the new RNs and the regular staff and was told the following:

Comments made from the new RNs:
- Do not feel they are viewed as competent RNs.
- Staff members are impatient with them and take over tasks instead of letting them learn the tasks.
- Unlicensed personnel do not come to them with patient problems.
- General comments are made that make them feel incompetent.
- Have even been told to "speak English" several times.
- Their names have been changed to names that the staff can easily pronounce.
- There are a couple of RNs and staff members who are sympathetic and helpful.

Comments made from the regular RNs and staff:
- Handoff reports are difficult to understand.
- Interactions with patients are minimal and not personal.
- They require a lot of guidance and leave many tasks for the other shifts.
- New RNs are afraid to approach physicians or to call physicians for orders.

1. List the primary issues as viewed by the new RNs.	2. List the primary issues as viewed by the regular RNs and staff.

Analyze the issues presented and list the management and cultural issues that need to be addressed.

Management-Related Issues/Needs	Culturally Related Issues/Needs

List management strategies that should be considered to address the issues presented:

_____

_____

_____

_____

_____

_____

_____

_____

_____

_____

_____

In the clinical setting, it is important to become aware of cultural communication (tone of voice, use of words, gestures, touch, nonverbal communication) with staff and peers.

With a partner, identify cultural beliefs and values seen among peers and staff in the clinical setting. Discuss clinical examples and the implications related to health care delivery.

Possible cultural beliefs and values:

INSTRUCTIONS: Circle the one best answer for each test question. Write your rationale for selecting the answer. To enhance your learning and test-taking skills, discuss your answer and rationale with a partner. The answer and the rationale can be found on the back of this page.

1. The nurse is demonstrating how to minimize occlusion of a feeding tube when administering medications. Which nursing intervention is most important to include in the demonstration?
   a. Withdraw any residual, give the medication, and flush with 30 mL of water.
   b. Flush the tube with 30 mL of water before and after giving the medication.
   c. Use 30 mL of lukewarm water to flush the tube after giving the medication.
   d. Inject 15 mL of air before and after giving the medication.

Rationale: _____
_____
_____
_____
_____

2. The client is discharged on phenytoin (Dilantin) 100 mg po q8h at 0800-1600-2400 and an antacid 30 mL prn. For effective drug administration, discharge instructions should include:
   a. Administer the phenytoin with a dose of antacid.
   b. Skip a dose of the phenytoin if the antacid is taken.
   c. Take half the dose of antacid if given with the phenytoin.
   d. Drink the antacid two hours before or after taking the phenytoin.

Rationale: _____
_____
_____
_____
_____

3. The client is receiving total parenteral nutrition through a single-lumen central catheter by infusion pump. Vancomycin 0.5 g in 100 mL 0.9% normal saline is ordered daily IVPB. To safely administer this IVPB, the nurse plans to:
   a. administer the IVPB through a Y-port tubing above the infusion pump.
   b. stop the total parenteral nutrition infusion for 30 minutes to infuse the IVPB.
   c. start a peripheral line for the IVPB.
   d. use a mini-drip tubing for the IVPB.

Rationale: _____
_____
_____
_____
_____

FIVE

ANSWER KEY FOR NCLEX EXAMINATION PREPARATION #1

HELPFUL HINTS: Read all test questions carefully. Identify key words in the question that will guide you in answering the question. In these test questions the **key words** to consider are **"most important," "effective drug administration,"** and **"safely."** Compare your rationale with the one in the test question.

1. The nurse is demonstrating how to minimize occlusion of a feeding tube when administering medications. Which nursing intervention is most important to include in the demonstration?
   a. Withdraw any residual, give the medication, and flush with 30 mL of water.
   b. Flush the tube with 30 mL of water before and after giving the medication.
   c. Use 30 mL of lukewarm water to flush the tube after giving the medication.
   d. Inject 15 mL of air before and after giving the medication.

   Rationale: The answer is (b). It is important to check the patency of the feeding tube before the administration of medications. Flushing the feeding tube after medication administration helps to clear the feeding tube. Options (a), (c), and (d) do not present the proper technique for administering medications through a feeding tube.

2. The client is discharged on phenytoin (Dilantin) 100 mg po q8h at 0800-1600-2400 and an antacid 30 mL prn. For effective drug administration, discharge instructions should include:
   a. Administer the phenytoin with a dose of antacid.
   b. Skip a dose of the phenytoin if the antacid is taken.
   c. Take half the dose of antacid if given with the phenytoin.
   d. Drink the antacid two hours before or after taking the phenytoin.

   Rationale: The answer is (d). Absorption of phenytoin may be decreased when it is taken with an antacid. Options (a) and (c) do not address the effects of an antacid on phenytoin. Drug therapy should not be altered; therefore option (b) is not correct.

3. The client is receiving total parenteral nutrition through a single-lumen central catheter by infusion pump. Vancomycin 0.5 g in 100 mL 0.9% normal saline is ordered daily IVPB. To safely administer this IVPB, the nurse plans to:
   a. administer the IVPB through a Y-port tubing above the infusion pump.
   b. stop the total parenteral nutrition infusion for 30 minutes to infuse the IVPB.
   c. start a peripheral line for the IVPB.
   d. use a mini-drip tubing for the IVPB.

   Rationale: The answer is (c). The IVPB should be administered via a separate IV line. Option (a) does not safely administer the IVPB because the total parenteral nutrition is continuously being infused. Option (b) indicates stopping the total parenteral nutrition, which may initiate a hypoglycemic reaction. Option (d) can be used but does not identify where the IVPB will be administered.

5-2 NCLEX EXAMINATION PREPARATION #2

INSTRUCTIONS: Circle the one best answer for each test question. Write your rationale for selecting the answer. To enhance your learning and test-taking skills, discuss your answer and rationale with a partner. The answer and the rationale can be found on the back of this page.

1. The nurse learns in report that the serum potassium level of a client is 5.5 mEq/L this morning. The client's physician is in surgery, so a message is left at the physician's office. The client is on the following medications at 0800: famotidine (Pepcid) 20 mg po and spironolactone (Aldactone) 50 mg po. Which action by the nurse is most appropriate?
   a. Hold the morning dose of famotidine until the physician returns the call.
   b. Hold the morning dose of spironolactone until the physician returns the call.
   c. Hold all the morning medications until the physician returns the call.
   d. Give all the morning medications as ordered.

   Rationale: _____
   _____
   _____
   _____
   _____

2. The nurse is caring for a client with diabetes mellitus type 2. The following medications are listed on the client's medication record: metformin (Glucophage) 0.5 g po bid and repaglinide (Prandin) 1 mg po with meals. The morning blood glucose fingerstick is 98 mg/dL. Which action by the nurse is most appropriate?
   a. Hold the morning po medications.
   b. Give the metformin but hold the repaglinide.
   c. Give the repaglinide but hold the metformin.
   d. Give the po medications as ordered.

   Rationale: _____
   _____
   _____
   _____
   _____

3. The client with end-stage renal disease is scheduled for hemodialysis in 2 hours. He has an (L) AV fistula and needs assistance with feeding. In delegating the care of the client to the nursing assistant, which nursing order is of priority?
   a. Feed the client first.
   b. Give all morning care before the dialysis.
   c. Take the blood pressure in the right arm.
   d. Gently feel for the thrill on the left arm.

   Rationale: _____
   _____
   _____
   _____
   _____

FIVE

ANSWER KEY FOR NCLEX EXAMINATION PREPARATION #2

HELPFUL HINTS: Read all test questions carefully. Identify key words in the question that will guide you in answering the question. In these test questions the **key words** to consider are **"most appropriate"** and **"priority."** Compare your rationale with the one in the test question.

1. The nurse learns in report that the serum potassium level of a client is 5.5 mEq/L this morning. The client's physician is in surgery, so a message is left at the physician's office. The client is on the following medications at 0800: famotidine (Pepcid) 20 mg po and spironolactone (Aldactone) 50 mg po. Which action by the nurse is most appropriate?
   a. Hold the morning dose of famotidine until the physician returns the call.
   b. Hold the morning dose of spironolactone until the physician returns the call.
   c. Hold all the morning medications until the physician returns the call.
   d. Give all the morning medications as ordered.

Rationale: The answer is (b). Spironolactone is a potassium-sparing diuretic. Because the morning serum K^+ level is high, the drug should be held and until further orders are obtained from the physician. Option (a) does not affect the potassium level. Options (c) and (d) do not correlate the effects of the specific drugs to the electrolyte value.

2. The nurse is caring for a client with diabetes mellitus type 2. The following medications are listed on the client's medication record: metformin (Glucophage) 0.5 g po bid and repaglinide (Prandin) 1 mg po with meals. The morning blood glucose fingerstick is 98 mg/dL. Which action by the nurse is most appropriate?
   a. Hold the morning po medications.
   b. Give the metformin but hold the repaglinide.
   c. Give the repaglinide but hold the metformin.
   d. Give the po medications as ordered.

Rationale: The answer is (d). The morning fingerstick result is within normal limits. Drug therapy should continue as ordered to maintain the blood glucose within normal limits. Options (a), (b), and (c) would not help the client remain in glycemic control.

3. The client with end-stage renal disease is scheduled for hemodialysis in 2 hours. He has an (L) AV fistula and needs assistance with feeding. In delegating the care of the client to the nursing assistant, which nursing order is of priority?
   a. Feed the client first.
   b. Give all morning care before the dialysis.
   c. Take the blood pressure in the right arm.
   d. Gently feel for the thrill on the left arm.

Rationale: The answer is (c). The AV fistula is the vascular access for the hemodialysis. Care must be taken not to occlude or cause trauma to the site. Options (a) and (b) are important but not the priority nursing order. Option (d) is part of the assessment process that is the responsibility of the professional nurse and should not be delegated.

INSTRUCTIONS: Circle the one best answer for each test question. Write your rationale for selecting the answer. To enhance your learning and test-taking skills, discuss your answer and rationale with a partner. The answer and the rationale can be found on the back of this page.

1. At 10:00 AM the nurse realizes that clonidine (Catapres) 0.1 mg po was administered to the wrong client at 9:00 AM. Which nursing action is of priority?
   a. Fill out an incident report.
   b. Notify the physician.
   c. Take the client's blood pressure.
   d. Take the vital signs of the client at noon.

Rationale: _____
_____
_____
_____
_____

2. A beta-blocking agent is added to the pharmacologic therapy of a client with heart failure. An expected therapeutic effect is:
   a. a decrease in complaints of fatigue.
   b. a decrease in the heart rate.
   c. an increase in blood pressure.
   d. an increase in diuresis.

Rationale: _____
_____
_____
_____
_____

3. The client is taking hydrochlorothiazide (Esidrix) 25 mg po daily and is started on the ACE inhibitor lisinopril (Zestril) 10 mg po daily. Which nursing intervention indicates the most appropriate follow-through action?
   a. Monitor the client's output.
   b. Assess the client for impaired skin integrity.
   c. Assess the client's cardiac rhythm.
   d. Monitor the client's blood pressure.

Rationale: _____
_____
_____
_____
_____

HELPFUL HINTS: Read all test questions carefully. Identify key words in the question that will guide you in answering the question. In these test questions the **key words** to consider are **"priority," "expected therapeutic effect,"** and **"most appropriate."** Compare your rationale with the one in the test question.

1. At 10:00 AM the nurse realizes that clonidine (Catapres) 0.1 mg po was administered to the wrong client at 9:00 AM. Which nursing action is of priority?
   a. Fill out an incident report.
   b. Notify the physician.
   c. Take the client's blood pressure.
   d. Take the vital signs of the client at noon.

Rationale: The answer is (c). Clonidine is an alpha-adrenergic agonist and blocking agent. After oral administration, clonidine begins to exert its effect within 1 hour. Option (a) is necessary, but assessing the client is priority. Option (b) is important, but it will be important to inform the physician of the current blood pressure. Option (d) is a good follow-up intervention but not the priority intervention.

2. A beta-blocking agent is added to the pharmacologic therapy of a client with heart failure. An expected therapeutic effect is:
   a. a decrease in complaints of fatigue.
   b. a decrease in the heart rate.
   c. an increase in blood pressure.
   d. an increase in diuresis.

Rationale: The answer is (b). Beta-blockers decrease the effects of epinephrine and norepinephrine. The physiologic effect is to decrease cardiac contractibility and workload. The client may have an increase, rather than a decrease, in fatigue after beginning therapy–option (a). Options (c) and (d) do not address the mechanism of action of beta-blockers.

3. The client is taking hydrochlorothiazide (Esidrix) 25 mg po daily and is started on the ACE inhibitor lisinopril (Zestril) 10 mg po daily. Which nursing intervention indicates the most appropriate follow-through action?
   a. Monitor the client's output.
   b. Assess the client for impaired skin integrity.
   c. Assess the client's cardiac rhythm.
   d. Monitor the client's blood pressure.

Rationale: The answer is (d). The drug combination indicates the primary use is for the antihypertensive effects. Blood pressure should be monitored before and after drug administration. Options (a), (b), and (c) do not address the effects of the combined drug therapy.

INSTRUCTIONS: Circle the one best answer for each test question. Write your rationale for selecting the answer. To enhance your learning and test-taking skills, discuss your answer and rationale with a partner. The answer and the rationale can be found on the back of this page.

1. The home health nurse visits a client who has a history of heart failure. The client is on enalapril, furosemide, and isosorbide. While talking with the client, the nurse notices that the client has a persistent dry, nonproductive cough. Which nursing action is most appropriate?
   a. Ask whether the client is taking any cough medicine.
   b. Encourage the client to increase fluid intake.
   c. Ask whether the client has had any chest pain.
   d. Notify the physician.

Rationale: _____
_____
_____
_____
_____

2. The nurse is providing discharge instructions to an elderly client taking the following oral medications: warfarin 5 mg daily, furosemide 20 mg daily, and digoxin 0.125 mg every other day. Which of the following is most important for the nurse to include in the instructions?
   a. "You can take the pills with meals."
   b. "Call the doctor if you notice any bruising."
   c. "Use a pill box to remind you of the medicines you need to take."
   d. "Take the furosemide in the morning so you can sleep at night."

Rationale: _____
_____
_____
_____
_____

3. The nurse is delegating the care of a client who is now stable after requiring a chest tube insertion for complications related to the insertion of a central subclavian line the night before. Which intervention is most important for the nurse to ask the nursing assistant to carry out?
   a. Count the respiratory rate for 1 full minute.
   b. Keep the client in high Fowler position.
   c. Encourage the client to cough and deep breathe.
   d. Ask the client to remain in bed while the chest tube is in place.

Rationale: _____
_____
_____
_____
_____

FIVE

ANSWER KEY FOR NCLEX EXAMINATION PREPARATION #4

HELPFUL HINTS: Read all test questions carefully. Identify key words in the question that will guide you in answering the question. In these test questions the **key words** to consider are **"most appropriate"** and **"most important."** Compare your rationale with the one in the test question.

1. The home health nurse visits a client who has a history of heart failure. The client is on enalapril, furosemide, and isosorbide. While talking with the client, the nurse notices that the client has a persistent dry, nonproductive cough. Which nursing action is most appropriate?
   a. Ask whether the client is taking any cough medicine.
   b. Encourage the client to increase fluid intake.
   c. Ask whether the client has had any chest pain.
   d. Notify the physician.

Rationale: The answer is (d). A dry, nonproductive cough is a side effect of ACE inhibitors such as enalapril. This may warrant a change in therapy. Options (a), (b), and (c) do not address this side effect.

2. The nurse is providing discharge instructions to an elderly client taking the following oral medications: warfarin 5 mg daily, furosemide 20 mg daily, and digoxin 0.125 mg every other day. Which of the following is most important for the nurse to include in the instructions?
   a. "You can take the pills with meals."
   b. "Call the doctor if you notice any bruising."
   c. "Use a pill box to remind you of the medicines you need to take."
   d. "Take the furosemide in the morning so you can sleep at night."

Rationale: The answer is (b). On the basis of this situation, it is most important to teach the client to recognize signs of excessive anticoagulation therapy. Options (a) and (d) are good but not the most important. Option (c) may not be the best because mixing digoxin with the other pills may be confusing for the elderly client if the digoxin needs to be held.

3. The nurse is delegating the care of a client who is now stable after requiring a chest tube insertion for complications related to the insertion of a central subclavian line the night before. Which intervention is most important for the nurse to ask the nursing assistant to carry out?
   a. Count the respiratory rate for 1 full minute.
   b. Keep the client in high Fowler position.
   c. Encourage the client to cough and deep breathe.
   d. Ask the client to remain in bed while the chest tube is in place.

Rationale: The answer is (c). Clients with chest tubes should be encouraged to cough and deep breathe to enhance lung reexpansion. Options (a) and (b) are good but not the most important. Option (d) is not appropriate, and, unless contraindicated, the client should be encouraged to ambulate.

5-5 NCLEX EXAMINATION PREPARATION #5

INSTRUCTIONS: Circle the one best answer for each test question. Write your rationale for selecting the answer. To enhance your learning and test-taking skills, discuss your answer and rationale with a partner. The answer and the rationale can be found on the back of this page.

1. The client is on a heparin infusion after being diagnosed with a venous thrombus in the right leg. To best monitor the effect of the heparin therapy, the nurse would:
   a. assess for signs and symptoms of bleeding.
   b. check the aPTT.
   c. monitor the PT.
   d. check the stool for occult blood.

Rationale: _____

_____

_____

_____

_____

2. The nurse is assigned to a client who is 4 days postop thoracic surgery and has a chest tube. The nurse learns in morning report that there has not been any drainage from the chest tube for the last 24 hours. In assessing the closed-chest drainage system, the nurse notes that there are no fluctuations in the water-seal chamber. The client's respirations are 22, unlabored. In planning the client care, the nurse would prepare:
   a. for possible chest tube removal.
   b. for replacement of the chest tube.
   c. to increase the suction to the drainage system.
   d. to disconnect the chest tube from the drainage system.

Rationale: _____

_____

_____

_____

_____

3. An elderly client, 1 day postop right hip surgery, is confused and restless this morning. The client is receiving oxygen via a nasal cannula, has a continuous IV to gravity, and is pulling at the right hip dressing. In planning the care of the client, it is most appropriate to initially assign the:
   a. staff RN to care for the client.
   b. nursing assistant to monitor the client and report changes.
   c. nursing assistant but have the RN check the client every hour.
   d. LVN/LPN to care for the client and assess for increased confusion.

Rationale: _____

_____

_____

_____

_____

ANSWER KEY FOR NCLEX EXAMINATION PREPARATION #5

HELPFUL HINTS: Read all test questions carefully. Identify key words in the question that will guide you in answering the question. In these test questions the **key words** to consider are **"best"** and **"planning the client care."** Compare your rationale with the one in the test question.

1. The client is on a heparin infusion after being diagnosed with a venous thrombus in the right leg. To best monitor the effect of the heparin therapy, the nurse would:
   a. assess for signs and symptoms of bleeding.
   b. check the aPTT.
   c. monitor the PT.
   d. check the stool for occult blood.

Rationale: The answer is (b). The aPTT (activated partial thromboplastin time) is used to monitor heparin therapy. Options (a) and (d) are good nursing interventions, but signs and symptoms are not the best indicators. Option (c) is mainly used to monitor warfarin therapy.

2. The nurse is assigned to a client who is 4 days postop thoracic surgery and has a chest tube. The nurse learns in morning report that there has not been any drainage from the chest tube for the last 24 hours. In assessing the closed-chest drainage system, the nurse notes that there are no fluctuations in the water-seal chamber. The client's respirations are 22, unlabored. In planning the client care, the nurse would prepare:
   a. for possible chest tube removal.
   b. for replacement of the chest tube.
   c. to increase the suction to the drainage system.
   d. to disconnect the chest tube from the drainage system.

Rationale: The answer is (a). The client is 4 days postop. Respiratory signs indicate normal progression of lung reexpansion. Assessment findings do not support option (b). Options (c) and (d) demonstrate a need to review chest tubes and the drainage system.

3. An elderly client, 1 day postop right hip surgery, is confused and restless this morning. The client is receiving oxygen via a nasal cannula, has a continuous IV to gravity, and is pulling at the right hip dressing. In planning the care of the client, it is most appropriate to initially assign the:
   a. staff RN to care for the client.
   b. nursing assistant to monitor the client and report changes.
   c. nursing assistant but have the RN check the client every hour.
   d. LVN/LPN to care for the client and assess for increased confusion.

Rationale: The answer is (a). Clients whose medical condition is unstable should be assigned to the RN. The RN is the most appropriate person to assess and monitor for changes. Options (b) and (c) are not appropriate for this client who is medically unstable. Option (d) is not appropriate because it is not in the LVN/LPN scope of practice to assess clients.

5-6 NCLEX EXAMINATION PREPARATION #6

INSTRUCTIONS: Circle the one best answer for each test question. Write your rationale for selecting the answer. To enhance your learning and test-taking skills, discuss your answer and rationale with a partner. The answer and the rationale can be found on the back of this page.

1. The client is being treated with continuous heparin infusion for a pulmonary embolus. The morning result of the activated partial thromboplastin time (aPTT) is 100 sec (control 30 sec). Which nursing intervention is of priority?
   a. Continue to monitor the client.
   b. Take the client's vital signs.
   c. Notify the physician.
   d. Check the previous result.

Rationale: _____

_____

_____

_____

_____

2. The nurse is caring for a client who has a chest tube connected to a closed-chest drainage system with suction. In assessing the water-seal chamber, the nurse notes constant bubbling. Which nursing intervention is most appropriate?
   a. Document the findings.
   b. Continue to monitor the client.
   c. Check the chest tube for air leaks.
   d. Decrease the amount of suction.

Rationale: _____

_____

_____

_____

_____

3. The nurse is totaling the chest tube output at 1400, the close of the shift. The chest tube drainage is at the 125 mL calibrated mark on the drainage device. The vertical tape along the side of the calibrated marks of the drainage device has a line drawn at 50 mL with the time of 0600. Which nursing intervention is most appropriate on the basis of this finding?
   a. Draw a line at 125 mL and indicate 1400.
   b. Document 125 mL as the output for the shift.
   c. Assess the suction chamber for patency.
   d. Strip or milk chest tube quickly for 5 to 10 seconds.

Rationale: _____

_____

_____

_____

_____

FIVE

ANSWER KEY FOR NCLEX EXAMINATION PREPARATION #6

HELPFUL HINTS: Read all test questions carefully. Identify key words in the question that will guide you in answering the question. In these test questions the **key words** to consider are **"priority"** and **"most appropriate."** Compare your rationale with the one in the test question.

1. The client is being treated with continuous heparin infusion for a pulmonary embolus. The morning result of the activated partial thromboplastin time (aPTT) is 100 sec (control 30 sec). Which nursing intervention is of priority?
   a. Continue to monitor the client.
   b. Take the client's vital signs.
   c. Notify the physician.
   d. Check the previous result.

Rationale: The answer is (c). The goal of heparin infusion is to maintain the activated partial thromboplastin time at 1.5 to 2, the normal range. The 100 sec result is a critical value, and the client is at risk for bleeding. Options (a), (b), and (d) are good nursing interventions but not the priority intervention.

2. The nurse is caring for a client who has a chest tube connected to a closed-chest drainage system with suction. In assessing the water-seal chamber, the nurse notes constant bubbling. Which nursing intervention is most appropriate?
   a. Document the findings.
   b. Continue to monitor the client.
   c. Check the chest tube for air leaks.
   d. Decrease the amount of suction.

Rationale: The answer is (c). Constant bubbling in the water-seal chamber indicates an air leak. Options (a) and (b) are good interventions but are not the most appropriate on the basis of the situation. Option (d) does not address the water-seal chamber.

3. The nurse is totaling the chest tube output at 1400, the close of the shift. The chest tube drainage is at the 125 mL calibrated mark on the drainage device. The vertical tape along the side of the calibrated marks of the drainage device has a line drawn at 50 mL with the time of 0600. Which nursing intervention is most appropriate on the basis of this finding?
   a. Draw a line at 125 mL and indicate 1400.
   b. Document 125 mL as the output for the shift.
   c. Assess the suction chamber for patency.
   d. Strip or milk chest tube quickly for 5 to 10 seconds.

Rationale: The answer is (a). The nurse monitors the chest tube drainage output by drawing a line at drainage level in the chamber at the end of the shift. Option (b) does not reflect the correct chest tube drainage for the shift, which is 75 mL. Option (c) is not an appropriate intervention, and option (d) is not standard nursing practice when caring for clients with chest tubes.

5-7 NCLEX EXAMINATION PREPARATION #7

INSTRUCTIONS: Circle the one best answer for each test question. Write your rationale for selecting the answer. To enhance your learning and test-taking skills, discuss your answer and rationale with a partner. The answer and the rationale can be found on the back of this page.

1. The nurse assesses the client who is 1 day postop transurethral resection of the prostate. He has not had any output from the urinary catheter for 2 hours. The client has an order for intermittent manual bladder irrigation. Which technique is best for the nurse to use to safely carry out this order?
   a. Irrigate with 50 mL of sterile water and aspirate an equal amount of fluid.
   b. Use clean technique and irrigate until the return is free of clots.
   c. Use sterile technique and irrigate with 50 mL of solution at a time.
   d. Start continuous bladder irrigation and infuse 200 mL over 30 minutes.

Rationale: _____
_____
_____
_____
_____

2. The client has just had a generalized tonic-clonic type seizure in bed. Which nursing intervention is of priority immediately after the seizure?
   a. Document the findings.
   b. Maintain a quiet environment.
   c. Reorient the client to the surroundings.
   d. Position the client in a side-lying position.

Rationale: _____
_____
_____
_____
_____

3. The nurse is assigned to a client who is 4 days postop right hip replacement. The nurse finds the client eating breakfast, sitting comfortably in a chair with the right leg crossed over the left leg. Which nursing intervention is of priority?
   a. Assess the right hip dressing.
   b. Assess the client's pain level.
   c. Check the quality of the pedal pulses of both feet.
   d. Instruct the client to keep both feet flat on the floor.

Rationale: _____
_____
_____
_____
_____

FIVE

ANSWER KEY FOR NCLEX EXAMINATION PREPARATION #7

HELPFUL HINTS: Read all test questions carefully. Identify key words in the question that will guide you in answering the question. In these test questions the **key words** to consider are **"best"** and **"priority."** Compare your rationale with the one in the test question.

1. The nurse assesses the client who is 1 day postop transurethral resection of the prostate. He has not had any output from the urinary catheter for 2 hours. The client has an order for intermittent manual bladder irrigation. Which technique is best for the nurse to use to safely carry out this order?
   a. Irrigate with 50 mL of sterile water and aspirate an equal amount of fluid.
   b. Use clean technique and irrigate until the return is free of clots.
   c. Use sterile technique and irrigate with 50 mL of solution at a time.
   d. Start continuous bladder irrigation and infuse 200 mL over 30 minutes.

   Rationale: The answer is (c). Bladder irrigation is always performed with sterile technique. Solution is gently introduced into the bladder during irrigation. Options (a), (b), and (d) do not describe how to safely and correctly carry out this technique.

2. The client has just had a generalized tonic-clonic type seizure in bed. Which nursing intervention is of priority immediately after the seizure?
   a. Document the findings.
   b. Maintain a quiet environment.
   c. Reorient the client to the surroundings.
   d. Position the client in a side-lying position.

   Rationale: The answer is (d). Aspiration is a concern after the seizure because the client will be lethargic and oral secretions will need to be suctioned and allowed to drain. Options (a), (b), and (c) are good interventions but are not priority.

3. The nurse is assigned to a client who is 4 days postop right hip replacement. The nurse finds the client eating breakfast, sitting comfortably in a chair with the right leg crossed over the left leg. Which nursing intervention is of priority?
   a. Assess the right hip dressing.
   b. Assess the client's pain level.
   c. Check the quality of the pedal pulses of both feet.
   d. Instruct the client to keep both feet flat on the floor.

   Rationale: The answer is (d). Crossing of the feet or legs after hip replacement may put undue tension on the operative hip and increase the risk of hip dislocation. Options (a) and (c) are good interventions but not the priority interventions. Option (b) is important; initial client observation indicates that client is eating and sitting comfortably.

5-8 NCLEX EXAMINATION PREPARATION #8

INSTRUCTIONS: Circle the one best answer for each test question. Write your rationale for selecting the answer. To enhance your learning and test-taking skills, discuss your answer and rationale with a partner. The answer and the rationale can be found on the back of this page.

1. The client is 4 days postop colon resection and has an NG tube to low continuous suction. The client tells the nurse that he is feeling nauseated and then vomits 100 mL of yellow-green drainage. The nurse's initial action is to:
   a. assess tube placement and patency.
   b. administer an antiemetic.
   c. pull out the NG tube.
   d. increase the NG tube suction to moderate.

Rationale: _____
_____
_____
_____
_____

2. The client has been on full-strength formula tube feeding at 60 mL/hr through the NG tube for 2 days. In delegating the care of the client, which directive, given to the nursing assistant, most indicates that the nurse is monitoring for tube feeding complications?
   a. "Let me know if the client has liquid bowel movements this shift."
   b. "Weigh the client on the stand-up scale as soon as report is over."
   c. "The client can sit in a chair for 30 minutes this morning."
   d. "Take the vital signs every 4 hours."

Rationale: _____
_____
_____
_____

3. The physician orders continuous PEG tube feedings at 50 mL/hr. After starting the tube feeding, it is most important for the nurse to initially plan to:
   a. assess bowel sounds every shift.
   b. take the vital signs q4h.
   c. monitor residual q4h.
   d. monitor the intake and output.

Rationale: _____
_____
_____
_____

ANSWER KEY FOR NCLEX EXAMINATION PREPARATION #8

HELPFUL HINTS: Read all test questions carefully. Identify key words in the question that will guide you in answering the question. In these test questions the **key words** to consider are **"initial," "most indicates,"** and **"most important."** Compare your rationale with the one in the test question.

1. The client is 4 days postop colon resection and has an NG tube to low continuous suction. The client tells the nurse that he is feeling nauseated and then vomits 100 mL of yellow-green drainage. The nurse's initial action is to:
   a. assess tube placement and patency.
   b. administer an antiemetic.
   c. pull out the NG tube.
   d. increase the NG tube suction to moderate.

Rationale: The answer is (a). It is important to check the placement and patency of the NG tube and ensure that the suction is working. Option (b) may be performed if the nausea and vomiting do not subside, but should not be the initial action. Options (c) and (d) do not help to solve the problem.

2. The client has been on full-strength formula tube feeding at 60 mL/hr through the NG tube for 2 days. In delegating the care of the client, which directive, given to the nursing assistant, most indicates that the nurse is monitoring for tube feeding complications?
   a. "Let me know if the client has liquid bowel movements this shift."
   b. "Weigh the client on the stand-up scale as soon as report is over."
   c. "The client can sit in a chair for 30 minutes this morning."
   d. "Take the vital signs every 4 hours."

Rationale: The answer is (a). Enteral feeding formulas can cause diarrhea. Option (b) helps to identify whether the client is gaining weight. Options (c) and (d) are directives that promote good nursing care, but they are not directly related to identifying the effects related to full strength formula tube feedings.

3. The physician orders continuous PEG tube feedings at 50 mL/hr. After starting the tube feeding, it is most important for the nurse to initially plan to:
   a. assess bowel sounds every shift.
   b. take the vital signs q4h.
   c. monitor residual q4h.
   d. monitor the intake and output.

Rationale: The answer is (c). Residual should be checked to ensure that the client is absorbing the tube feeding. Residuals greater than 200 mL, or as ordered by physician, increase the client's risk for vomiting and aspiration. Options (a), (b), and (d) are important but are not the most important.

6-1 QUALITY NURSING PRACTICE SITUATION #1 (POSTSURGICAL PATIENT)

Nursing Care Plan		
Lab/Diagnostic Tests	**Medications**	
ECG ☑	Ketorolac 10 mg IM q6h ×24 hr Acetaminophen #3 tab i po q3h prn pain Metoclopramide 10 mg IVP q6h prn N/V	Diet: Clear liquid - DAT
	Indwelling urinary catheter	VS q4h Antiembolic stockings Seq. compression device	Ambulate with assistance Incentive spirometer q2h
IV Fluids: 1 L lactated Ringer's q8h		
Name: CJ Age: 60 Full code	Dx: Prostate cancer Surg: da Vinci laparoscopic radical prostatectomy	

Morning handoff report: "The patient is 1 day postop. He was possibly being discharged today, but he had some chest pain last night and I heard fine crackles on the right lower lung base. Bowel sounds are faint in the four quadrants. Vital signs are stable. Pain level 2. The urinary catheter is patent, draining blood-tinged urine. Please encourage the patient to use the incentive spirometer and have him ambulate more today. An ECG was done last night. His doctor will be in sometime this morning."

Using Nursing Knowledge

Based on the morning handoff report and the nursing care plan, answer the following:
• List assessment priorities:

_____

_____

• Identify the priorities of the plan of care for the morning:

_____

• List signs and symptoms that might indicate possible complications that the nurse should monitor and include in the plan of care:

_____

_____

Using Leadership Skills

Consider the scope of practice and then determine the nursing interventions that may be delegated to the:

LVN/LPN:

_____

_____

_____

_____

Unlicensed personnel:

_____

_____

_____

Evidence-Based Practice
Use appropriate resources to answer the following question:
In clients who have a radical prostatectomy, how effective is the da Vinci surgical method in enhancing postop recovery compared to clients who have a transurethral resection of the prostate?

_____

_____

SIX

Review the following diagram, "Caring for the Whole Person." Use the boxes to:
1. Identify <u>**actual and potential**</u> concerns related to the social needs of the client.
2. Identify the **physiologic** needs at discharge.
3. List **individual considerations** for the client on discharge.

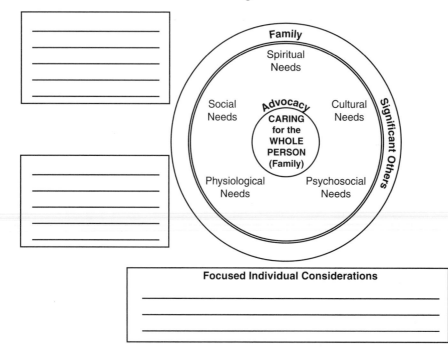

Focused Individual Considerations

⚡ **Integrated Learning Activity:** With a partner, use the textbooks and information from appropriate websites to answer and complete the possible discharge instructions for the client:

Possible discharge instructions:

Regarding Urinary Catheter:	
Discharge Medications:	
Activity:	
Follow-up Visit:	
Potential Complications:	

6-2 QUALITY NURSING PRACTICE SITUATION #2 (CARING AND ADVOCACY)

Nursing Care Plan		
Lab/Diagnostic Tests	**Medications**	
FBG in AM Electrolyte panel in AM UA ☐	Lorazepam 0.5 mg IV stat O$_2$ per NC @ 3 L/min	Diet: Mech soft NPO p̄ midnight VS, pulse ox q4h and prn I & O q shift Bed rest
IV Fluids: 1 L Normal Saline 0.9% at 50 mL/hr		
Name: SP Age: 75	Full code	Dx: Acute confusion

Evening Handoff Report at 2300: "The client was admitted from the emergency department around 1900. The wife says that she noticed that her husband started to get confused last evening. The wife, who is 70 yrs old, has been with him all day and looks very tired. She is waiting for her son to pick her up but does not really want to leave her husband. She says they have been married 50 years and they rarely have been separated from each other. The admitting orders are on the chart. I gave him lorazepam IV for restlessness at 2100. The wife says he has been taking zolpidem for sleep. You might want to call the doctor for an order of zolpidem if the lorazepam does not calm him down. The latest VS are T 99.6° F, P 92 irregular, R 18 shallow, BP 136/90, pulse ox 94% on oxygen at 3 L/min. Unable to determine if the patient is having pain since he does not respond appropriately to the pain assessment scale."

Using Nursing Knowledge

Based on the evening report and nursing care plan, answer the following:
- List assessment priorities:

  _____
  _____

- Identify the priorities of the plan of care for the shift:

  _____
  _____
  _____
  _____

- List signs and symptoms that might indicate possible complications that the nurse should monitor and include in the plan of care:

  _____
  _____

Using Leadership Skills

Consider the scope of practice, then determine the nursing interventions that may be delegated for this client to the:

LVN/LPN:

_____
_____
_____
_____

Unlicensed personnel:

_____
_____
_____
_____

Evidence-Based Practice
Use appropriate resources to answer the following question:
In elderly clients age 75 years and older, is lorazepam effective in decreasing anxiety and restlessness?
_____
_____

SIX

Review the following diagram, "Caring for the Whole Person." Use the boxes to:
1. Identify <u>**actual and potential**</u> **physiologic** concerns related to the care of the client.
2. Identify the <u>**actual or potential**</u> **psychosocial** concerns expressed by the <u>wife</u>.
3. List **individual considerations** for the care of the client.

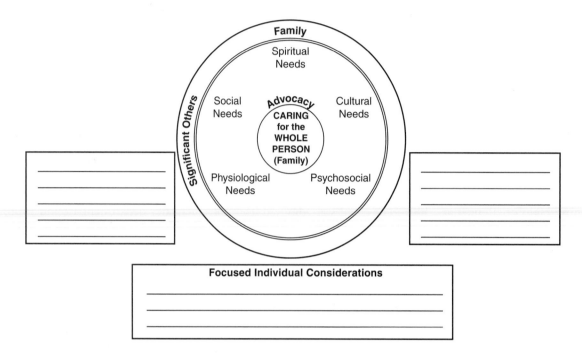

Focused Individual Considerations

_____

_____

_____

Integrated Learning Activity: With a partner, use the following part of the clinical situation to write possible therapeutic communication statements that demonstrate caring and advocacy:

The wife, who is 70 years old, has been with him all day and looks very tired. She is waiting for her son to pick her up but does not really want to leave her husband. She says they have been married 50 years and they rarely have been separated from each other.

Write possible therapeutic communication statements that demonstrate **caring:**

_____

_____

_____

_____

_____

_____

_____

Write a possible therapeutic communication statement that demonstrates **advocacy:**

_____

_____

_____

_____

6-3 QUALITY NURSING PRACTICE SITUATION #3 (ADVERSE CLIENT OUTCOME)

Nursing Care Plan		
Medications		
FSBG qAM & qPM (Call MD if greater than 150 mg/dL) O₂ per NC @ 3 L/min prn	Amlodipine 5 mg po daily Cimetidine 400 mg po QID Glyburide 2.5 mg po daily Nitroglycerin 0.4 mg SL i tab q5min ×3 prn chest pain	Diet: 1800 ADA VS q4h I & O Up in chair tid Antiembolic hose
Saline Lock Flush with NS q shift		
Name: RA Age: 60	Full code	Dx: Pneumonia, hypertension Hx of CAD, unstable angina DM type 2

Handoff Report at 0700: "The client had a restful night. He says he is going home this morning. His lungs are clear and the vital signs are stable with a BP of 140/88. He complained of some indigestion a little while ago, so I gave the cimetidine early. Aside from his routine medications and removal of his saline lock on discharge, he is ready to go."

Progression of Adverse Outcome

- After report the RN visits the client and asks the client whether the cimetidine has helped him. The client says it was just given to him so that it will take a few more minutes for the drug to work. He asks for the emesis basin "just in case."
- The RN asks the unlicensed assistant to take the pulse and BP because the client is diaphoretic. Dynamap readings indicate an increase in pulse and a BP of 120/70.
- The RN asks the LVN to start the oxygen and asks the CNA to take vital signs q5min.
- The RN goes to call the physician.
- Ten minutes later the LVN calls a code. After 30 minutes of CPR the client is pronounced dead.

Using Leadership Skills

List the current needs that are associated with the care of the family experiencing the death of a loved one:

- Prepare for family visit (Who should be involved?)
  _____
- Postdeath care can be done by:
  _____
- Notify pastoral care (Who should notify?)
  _____
- Document (Who should document?)
  _____

Evaluate the situation:
What could have been done differently?
_____
_____
_____
_____

Evidence-Based Practice

Use appropriate resources to answer the following question:
In acute care settings that have rapid response teams, are nursing staff from noncritical care units consistently utilizing the rapid response team for patients who are clinically deteriorating?
_____
_____
_____
_____

SIX

Review the following diagram, "Caring for the Whole Person." Use the boxes to:

1. Identify **actual and potential** psychosocial needs for the **family** related to the unexpected death of the client.
2. List **individual considerations** for the postdeath care of the client.

Focused Individual Considerations

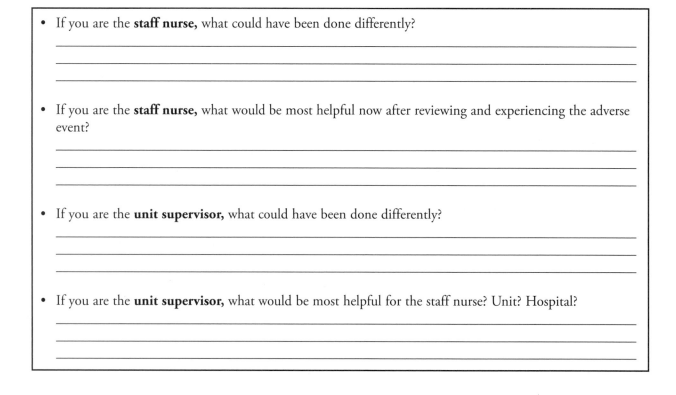

⚡ **Integrated Learning Activity:** With a partner, reread the situation. Discuss and answer the following:

- If you are the **staff nurse,** what could have been done differently?

- If you are the **staff nurse,** what would be most helpful now after reviewing and experiencing the adverse event?

- If you are the **unit supervisor,** what could have been done differently?

- If you are the **unit supervisor,** what would be most helpful for the staff nurse? Unit? Hospital?

7-1 WORKING WITH PHARMACOLOGY #1

Instructions: Read the mini scenario, and from your knowledge of pharmacology, fill in the drug classification for the drug identified in the scenario. All of the listed **side effects/adverse effects** are associated with the drug. Research the side effect/adverse effect that is highlighted with a (●) using appropriate resources.

- Write the research findings.
- Identify patient instructions related to this drug therapy.

The nurse is caring for a patient who has been taking atorvastatin (Lipitor) 20 mg po BID for 2 months to lower cholesterol levels. **Drug Classification:**	Side effects/adverse effects of this drug: • Headache • Dizziness • Muscle pain ● • Abdominal cramps • Skin rash	Research findings:
The nurse is caring for a patient who has been taking propranolol (Inderal) 80 mg po q8h to control an irregular heartbeat. **Drug Classification:**	Side effects/adverse effects of this drug: • Slow pulse ● • Dizziness • Weakness • Impotence • Skin rash	Research findings:
The nurse is caring for a patient who has been taking phenytoin (Dilantin) 200 mg po q8h for a seizure disorder. **Drug Classification:**	Side effects/adverse effects of this drug: • Diplopia • Nystagmus • Weight loss • Swollen gums • Agranulocytosis ●	Research findings:

SEVEN

7-2 WORKING WITH PHARMACOLOGY #2

Instructions: Read the mini scenario, and from your knowledge of pharmacology, fill in the drug classification for the drug identified in the scenario. All of the listed **side effects/adverse effects** are associated with the drug. Research the side effect/adverse effect that is highlighted with a (●) using appropriate resources.
- Write the research findings.
- Identify patient instructions related to this drug therapy.

The nurse is assessing a patient who has been taking prednisone 10 mg po daily for 2 months for Crohn disease. **Drug Classification:**	**Side effects/adverse effects of this drug:** • Mood swings • Ecchymosis • Anorexia • Stomach pain ● • Restlessness	**Research findings:**
The nurse is administering ketorolac (Toradol) 10 mg IM q6h to a postsurgical patient. **Drug Classification:**	**Side effects/adverse effects of this drug:** • Drowsiness • Paresthesia • Abdominal pain ● • Dyspepsia • Urinary frequency	**Research findings:**
The nurse is assessing a patient who is on clopidogrel (Plavix) 75 mg po daily after suffering a recent stroke. **Drug Classification:**	**Side effects/adverse effects of this drug:** • Nose bleed • Neutropenia ● • Depression • Headache • Diarrhea	**Research findings:**

7-3 WORKING WITH PHARMACOLOGY #3

Instructions: Read the mini scenario, and from your knowledge of pharmacology, fill in the drug classification for the drug identified in the scenario. All of the listed **side effects/adverse effects** are associated with the drug. Research the side effect/adverse effect that is highlighted with a (●) using appropriate resources.
- Write the research findings.
- Identify patient instructions related to this drug therapy.

The nurse administers lorazepam (Ativan) 4 mg IVP as a preop medication to a patient. **Drug Classification:**	**Side effects/adverse effects of this drug:** • Dizziness • Dyspnea ● • Lethargy • Depression • Drowsiness	**Research findings:**
The nurse is preparing the 0900 dose of captopril (Capoten) 50 mg po for the patient diagnosed with heart failure. **Drug Classification:**	**Side effects/adverse effects of this drug:** • Fatigue • Headache • Nonproductive cough • Neutropenia ● • Dizziness	**Research findings:**
The nurse is assessing a patient who is on digoxin (Lanoxin) 0.25 mg po daily for a patient who has atrial fibrillation. **Drug Classification:**	**Side effects/adverse effects of this drug:** • Dysrhythmia ● • Fatigue • Yellow vision • Abdominal pain • Headache	**Research findings:**

SEVEN

7-4 WORKING WITH PHARMACOLOGY #4

Instructions: Read the mini scenario, and from your knowledge of pharmacology, fill in the drug classification for the drug identified in the scenario. All of the listed **side effects/adverse effects** are associated with the drug. Research the side effect/adverse effect that is highlighted with a (●) using appropriate resources.

- Write the research findings.
- Identify patient instructions related to this drug therapy.

The nurse is administering **levofloxacin (Levaquin) 500 mg IVPB daily to a patient post-operatively.** **Drug Classification:**	Side effects/adverse effects of this drug: • Dizziness • Insomnia • Abdominal pain • Diarrhea • Tendon pain ●	Research findings:

The nurse is teaching a patient how to use a metaproterenol sulfate (Alupent) inhaler and signs and symptoms related to use. **Drug Classification:**	Side effects/adverse effects of this drug: • Nervousness • Headache • Difficulty breathing ● • Fine hand tremors • Restlessness	Research findings:

The patient is started on vancomycin 500 mg in 100 mL 0.9% normal saline IVPB daily. **Drug Classification:**	Side effects/adverse effects of this drug: • Phlebitis • Flushing of face/torso ● • Nausea • Headache • Diarrhea	Research findings:

7-5 WORKING WITH DECISION MAKING

Instructions: Read the mini scenario found in the box. Then decide whether the clinical decision, action, or intervention made by the nurse was appropriate. Provide a rationale for your decision.

Situation #1	Clinical Decision/Action/Intervention
The nurse is caring for a patient who has been diagnosed with diabetes mellitus type 1. The patient is started on insulin glargine 26 units daily in the evening and a correction bolus insulin scale (sliding scale) with regular insulin (Humulin R). The nurse provides the following instructions to the patient: 1. Insulin glargine is a long-acting insulin that is administered once a day, usually in the evening. 2. Regular insulin may be combined with insulin glargine in the same insulin syringe if your fingerstick blood glucose results indicate the need for regular bolus insulin coverage.	☐ **Appropriate** ☐ **Not Appropriate** **Rationale:**

Situation #2	Clinical Decision/Action/Intervention
The nurse is caring for a patient diagnosed with a DVT. An IV of 1000 mL 0.9% NS with heparin 20,000 units is started and the physician orders for the patient to receive 500 units of heparin per hour. The nurse sets the IV pump at 32 mL/hr. Has the nurse carried out the order correctly?	☐ **Appropriate** ☐ **Not Appropriate** **Rationale:**

Situation #3	Clinical Decision/Action/Intervention
The RN is working with a staff LVN during the weekend. Throughout the shift, the RN delegates the following nursing interventions to the LVN: 1. Monitor a blood transfusion 2. Start an IV of lactated Ringer's solution 3. Collect a sterile UA specimen via a straight catheterization 4. Admit a new patient 5. Administer nitroglycerin SL to a patient experiencing angina	☐ **Appropriate** ☐ **Not Appropriate** **Rationale:**

SEVEN

7-6 WORKING WITH PRIORITY SETTING

Instructions: Read the Nursing Kardex (Rand) and the Nursing Notes from the night shift on client RM.

Diagnostic Tests	Routine Medications	
Na⁺, K⁺, Cl⁻, BUN	Furosemide 20 mg IVP 0900	Diet: 1800 Cal ADA NAS
CBC today (10/8)	Metformin 500 mg po BID	Bed rest with BRP
FBG today (10/8)	Docusate 100 mg po qAM Temazepam 7.5 mg po tab i at bedtime if needed	LBM: 10/06 VS routine
IVP today (10/8)	Saline lock inserted 10/05	Fingerstick BS qAM (0730) & qPM (1700)

	Humulin R insulin sliding scale:
	  200-175 give 4 units Humulin R insulin
	  174-150 give 2 units Humulin R insulin
	  149-125 no insulin
		I & O
		Chg Ⓛ leg dressing q shift
		Elevate leg on pillow

Pt. Name: RM	Age: 66 Admitted: 10/4 Rm: 255	Dx: Cellulitis left leg/DM type 2

Date	Time	Nurse's Notes
10/08	0100	Awake, states is worried about the infection in his leg. Left leg elevated on pillow. Dressing dry and intact, no drainage noted. Requested sleeping medication. Medicated with temazepam 7.5 mg.---N. Nurse RN
	0200	Sleeping--N. Nurse RN
	0600	Awake, small amount of serosanguineous drainage noted on dressing. c/o leg pain 5/10 on the pain scale, states "wants to wait to see if the pain goes away in a few minutes." Fasting blood glucose was drawn this morning.--N. Nurse RN

Instructions: Based on your evaluation of the Nursing Kardex and the Nursing Notes, (1) complete the clinical worksheet with your notes for the required care and, (2) list your priority nursing actions.

Clinical Worksheet	List Priority Nursing Actions
Pt. Name: _____ Room: _____ Dx: _____ VS: _____ at _____ Drg chg ( ) Saline lock ( ) I & O ( ) Elevate leg on pillow ( ) Medications: _____ _____ _____ _____ _____ _____	

APPENDIX A

LIST OF ABBREVIATIONS

ac	=	before meals
BUN	=	blood urea nitrogen
BM	=	bowel movement
BR	=	bed rest
Client	=	patient
CBC	=	complete blood count
Dx	=	diagnosis
ECG	=	electrocardiogram
FBG	=	fasting blood glucose
I & O	=	intake and output
Kardex	=	Rand/Patient Summary Report
NP	=	nasal prongs (same as nasal cannula = NC)
N/V	=	nausea/vomiting
NPO	=	nothing by mouth
OGTT	=	oral glucose tolerance test
PCA	=	patient-controlled analgesia
PT	=	protime
UA	=	urinalysis
VS	=	vital signs (T - P - R - B/P and pain level)
T	=	temperature
P	=	pulse
R	=	respirations
BP	=	blood pressure
Pulse ox	=	pulse oximetry
OOB	=	out of bed
ROM	=	range of motion

APPENDIX B

LIST OF WORDS AND PHRASES COMMONLY USED IN THE BOOK AND THEIR INTENDED MEANINGS

Assessment finding	=	presenting sign, symptom, laboratory data, complaint *Example:* Which assessment finding is of most concern?
Correction bolus insulin scale	=	sliding scale
Document the findings	=	to chart assessment data in the client's chart or to enter the assessment data in the computer program
Expected findings	=	assessment findings/lab data that are associated with the illness or diagnosis *Example:* A client has a hay fever allergy. ***Expected findings:*** watery, itchy eyes, clear mucus, sneezing *Example:* A client has anemia. ***Expected findings:*** decreased hemoglobin and hematocrit; serum Hgb and Hct below the normal range
Expected outcome	=	the desired outcome based on the implementation of appropriate interventions
Focused assessment	=	the signs and symptoms associated with the medical diagnosis or with the acute illness/condition
Kardex (Rand)	=	Patient Summary Report; contains the overview of current treatments, medications, diet, lab/diagnostic tests orders and specific interventions for the patient
Of priority	=	the sign/symptom/intervention that is of most concern *Example:* Which intervention is of priority . . .
Most effective	=	most appropriate for the situation *Example:* The most effective infection control method . . .
To effectively	=	to appropriately *Example:* To effectively use the incentive spirometer . . .
To implement	=	to put into action; to carry out *Example:* To implement this order effectively . . .
Predisposed	=	at risk or likely to develop *Example:* A client who smokes is predisposed to developing adverse lung conditions
The primary purpose	=	the most important reason or the primary reason *Example:* The primary purpose of the . . .